LIVING INTO THE 100S

════ WOW! ════

BY IRIS M. FORD

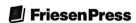 **FriesenPress**

Suite 300 - 990 Fort St
Victoria, BC, Canada, V8V 3K2
www.friesenpress.com

Copyright © 2015 by Iris M. Ford
First Edition — 2015

ISBN
978-1-4602-6205-4 (Hardcover)
978-1-4602-6206-1 (Paperback)
978-1-4602-6207-8 (eBook)

1. Self-Help, Aging

Distributed to the trade by The Ingram Book Company

LIVING INTO THE 100S

— WOW! —

TABLE OF CONTENTS

APPRECIATIONS

*There are so many people who have shared their
life stories in this book.
I am very pleased to welcome them as I share
their stories of how real
oldies; eighty, ninety and one hundred
cope. You will be amazed.*

*Most do not want their last names used so I will
just use first names
as I reach out to them in humble gratitude.
Dolly, Laurette, Beppie, Hilmer, Monica, Hazel
and David,
Betty, Gilbert, Elaine, Ruth,
Dorothy, and Raymonde.*

*THANK YOU FOR SHARING YOUR LIFE
STORIES.
GOD BLESS YOU.*

I am also very grateful to Ruth McCowan, who edited this manuscript for me and wrote the chapter on dementia. Thank you, Ruth.

INTRODUCTION

I'm a retired minister of the Presbyterian Church, and as one of the first female ministers in my denomination, I have always had a great interest in sharing my life story. As I enter my eighties, many of my friends are in their nineties, and one of them is even in her hundreds. Living here by the sea on lovely Vancouver Island, I spend a lot of time thinking about what aging really means.

I was talking with a friend the other day and sharing some memories from our childhood that would shock children if they heard them today. Childhood back several generations was often harshly disciplined. Mine? Yes. There was a time when my dad took a rod as his spanking device. I recall Dad taking me to the backyard and whipping me for some reason. What I had done escapes me. All I remember was the distrust it gave me towards a lot of things. My dad was not an angry man. He was just following my mother's orders.

What had I done? I don't remember but my mother used to hit us regularly with a stick she cut down from the cherry tree in the back yard. When we wanted to get her to calm down we hid the stick and by the time she had cut down a new one she had calmed down. Dad never seemed angry but Mother was always angry for some reason. We were not bad kids. It was the way discipline was carried out back then. If children were threatened by that kind of discipline today, they wouldn't believe it, they would just laugh and walk away. It is against the law now and looked on as mistreating the child.

Another friend told me of how as children they were disciplined in school way back in the early 1900s. My friend and another girl were sitting together and the other child was acting up. Finally, the male teacher took the rod and went to hit her with it but missed and hit my friend instead. It left a big welt and even though the teacher apologized later, the pain remained with her. As she looks back she told me that she always hated school.

Today I ask: How have we gone from cruel discipline back in our childhoods to no discipline worth mentioning today? What is good discipline? How do children grow up appreciating themselves, honouring their gifts, and calmly reaching out to others, feeling loved and secure? How has cruel discipline affected us as we have grown up? What has the negative influence done to our self-respect? Has it in any way affected how we have grown through the years, hindering us from reaching eighty, ninety, and even a hundred? What will children go through during these next hundred years? Is there a lack of discipline now as society goes the other way completely?

When I consider how I feel today, looking at my present day adulthood stance, I admit that I have always had an inner calm, helping me stand firm yet kind as I reached adulthood. This is especially true as I went into the ministry, where I was, in many incidences, the first woman minister people had ever met. Life back then and through to the present, has changed so much. Did I accept myself? I really had to believe in myself in order to preach to others in love and understanding. God's love must have had a lot to do with my ability to stand before others in faith and with joy, instead of with criticism and fear.

As people share their stories with me in this book, few have included the negative memories, and few have looked honestly at their childhoods with understanding eyes. Some have though and the difference is noticeable. They have reached their nineties, living without self-criticism, reaching out to others in love and with understanding. To live out their years means to accept self with its faults and sad memories.

Welcome to the journey to a hundred.

CHAPTER ONE

—

How Our World Has Changed

When I look back on my own childhood, and I am only eighty-two, I am amazed at how this world has changed during the last hundred years. It reminds me that big changes have taken place throughout the years during which we have grown up. This book does not look for reasons why, but is meant just to remind us of where the world was a hundred years ago. Oh boy, how everything has changed! The western world has come a long way, really fast. It is a little scary when we think of the future our grandchildren and great-grandchildren will be living through. What will this world be like a hundred years from now? I am thankful I lived in the century I did. I went through some really hard times though, with little acceptance of women in the working world. Yes, I was only the twentieth woman to be ordained as a minister in our denomination. Everywhere I went, people were curious and doubtful.

I think ahead with trepidation now. Few of us can recall what the world was like a hundred years ago but I know it was very different from today. Friends tell me what it was like back then in Scotland as many people have immigrated to Canada from the 'old' world and they are all around here. Liz, a good friend, describes her family's house back then. It was one big room with everything in it, including what we would call the kitchen area, living room, and dining room. It was just one large room!

In 1927, Liz was born in that old, one-room house with a district nurse to aid her birth. The bed was in a side alcove with a curtain hiding the exciting delivery. There were three other bed alcoves in along the wall. It had a kitchen table, four chairs, and a battery-powered radio as there was no electricity. Liz's mother cooked on a gas stove and the gas was piped in to the mantle on the chimney and had to be turned on.

Liz's memories cover everything in that old house until 1931. Her brother was also born there in the covered bed alcove. There were no phones and no cars. They used a horse and buggy to get around to the local grocery store. Each week, fruits, vegetables, fish, and milk were delivered by horse and buggy to the houses on their street. Everything was within walking distance, even the church. My friend started kindergarten at age five. She had cousins living close by and had plenty of friends to play with. The lavatory was outside. There was no running water so they were bathed once a week in a movable bathtub. Water had to be brought in from an outside tap and there was no privacy. What did it feel like to have friends and family so close? Wonderful!

In 1939, the family moved to a larger house where there was running water and electricity. The children played outside mostly. They played peeves, which involved making drawings on the road. They also played with spinning tops, Snakes and Ladders, and Luda, which was a board game that could be played inside on the table. The whole family would play that one together.

There were no TVs back then and the family spent the time we so carelessly waste today, by playing together. There was so much family interaction back then compared with today. The girls went to Brownies at age five to twelve, then to Girl Guides. Sunday school was Sunday afternoon. "We had to walk to church," Liz told me, and later she was a Sunday school teacher. The cousins and family members were all close by. Her cousin was her inseparable friend and they are on the phone to this day. Their health all seemed good as they never heard the cancer word back then. Everybody was healthy and happy. Liz's grandma died at seventy-six and her dad's mom was eighty when she died. The family had a lot of interaction together. As the family members separated and moved away, many came to Canada. No one seems to have experienced loneliness or separation feelings as everyone's lives were full of companionship and family support. They felt wanted and needed and they share those feelings with others today.

As I look at life in this modern age I am wondering how people will manage through today's challenges and on through the future generations. Families grow up not even knowing the family next door. There is separation anxiety all round and it will get even worse as iPods etc. separate us from personal contact. How will relationships be nurtured in the lives of our grandchildren these days? What will the next hundred years offer that will nurture the best in the human spirit?

One great memory I have from my own childhood in Bermuda is being driven home in a horse and carriage as there were no cars on the Island back then. We were all tired from spending the day at the beach and were sound asleep in the carriage being led home safely by the horse. I am wondering now if the present generations are like us; in the carriage being safely led home, but really not very aware of what is going on around them. We have our memories but what is being done today to encourage a better lifestyle in the present generation; one that can take our grandchildren and our great-grandchildren safely into the next hundred years? Or are we all asleep? What are you doing to help others cope as they age?

Dolly, an old friend of mine, shared her experiences with me. Dolly comments on what she is doing each week to help others cope as they age. Her words are few but profound.

"I do my level best to try to live by the Golden Rule if I can. I call widows and the lonely every day to see if they are OK. I send all kinds of cards out to them when there is a need. I volunteer at the Breithaupt Centre for the City of Kitchener. I try to help people any way I can and I also drive them around. I listen to people on the phone for hours as they unload their problems, and I try to counter-act it with good advice and an appropriate Bible verse. I have also given my little rescue doggie a good home.

"I am so very thankful and blest that I have very good friends and neighbours who look out for me. I enjoy my family when I can see them. Sometimes I do wonder why I'm still here. You asked how old I am – I am now eighty-six. I do not do as much at church any more, but I do send birthday cards to our seniors. This does not cover my life story but it is where I am at now, and I thank God for bringing me to this spot as He shows me how to use my time."

CHAPTER TWO

—

Looking Forward To Being 100

"You are going to call your book that?" people say. "Who is looking forward to being a hundred? You are talking nonsense."

Most people I have interviewed say, "I would rather be dead and never reach a hundred." So why do some reach it or did they not have a choice? I am now eighty-two years old and what do I look forward to – going beyond ninety? Really? I am already aching in most of my body, what with bad hips, high blood pressure, and bad eyesight. It will probably get worse.

Do I really think life at ninety and beyond would be joyous and beneficial? I wonder. One lady in her hundreds seemed to have a spark in her eyes when she was talking with me. But on another day the spark was gone and she complained that she was confused and not able to talk straight that day. She even asked me to pray for her. Will prayer help those waiting to die? What if the sufferer doesn't believe in God and never thought about meeting Jesus Christ? What could I say to encourage her? Someone help me here. I don't have an answer and I doubt whether I will have an answer by the end of this book unless God shows up.

Does this honesty grab you? Would you rather die young than live to an "old" age? What if your body disagreed and kept you going? Could you do anything in those final years that would be worthwhile and give you a reason for being still on this earth? What if God gave you an inner spark? Could you tell others what it means? Does God have anything to do with it?

I have spent many months researching this book, but this is all I have and it feels like it is not enough. The final decision is up to us, and our families too, if they live close by. We must go on alone if we have to.

I spent the last year and a half sitting beside my dear friend who has been suffering from dementia. I watched her die but she was too out of it mentally to know that was what was happening. We had spent the last fifteen years in a Roadtrek recreational vehicle travelling all over the place, having a wonderful retirement. She was encouraging me to come with her (on another trip) but I could not. She had to go on this trip alone.

Dying is the final journey and one has to go through it alone but I believe that Jesus meets us on the other side. You and I have to leave earth alone on the final journey of life – death. It is scary, right?

Here in this book we can explore together the many sides to aging. Please be patient with me as the road ahead is rocky, and few people have the words to put understanding on the trip ahead through life. Let's try! Let's look at ages eighty, ninety, and a hundred and ask each other: What are the truths that make the road ahead less awkward? What would help the loneliness and make the suffering bearable? When the way looks rough, let's try to understand each other for we all go through it sooner or later. I look forward to meeting many of you as we all travel this final road. Many have given me their life stories, which I will put in this book; chapter by chapter; story by story. They are all fascinating, but is there anything that stands out to explain their long lives?

When I look at my own life, several things stand out that may well have fashioned my life, since that skill or interest stayed with my brain. Music is one. I learned to play the piano at age nine, and the ability to sight-read music has stayed with me, enabling me to play the organ even now at age eighty-two. I can sight-read anything. It is as if my brain has stored the information. Other researchers suggest that in the senior years we should learn a new language to stir the brain to remember and recall something new and challenging. How much of a challenge do you face each day now that you are in your nineties or close to it?

Other writers suggest that we need to spend more time readying our brains for the future challenges. What about spending more time on meditation, or more time praying to God for His help? Why not spend more time thinking in a way that turns us away from self to reach out to others? Evidently people who volunteer and help others live beneficial lives live longer than most people in today's society. Sadly, in today's society most are working really hard to make a buck and they forget other people's needs. This is a busy society and is very tired and exhausted. I wonder how long you will live, friend. How long will I live? Will anyone care?

Here is the life story of a woman in her hundreds. Look for a spark and look for a desire to help others. What do you think is her secret?

LAURETTE'S LIFE STORY AT AGE 105

It was a beautiful, sunny Saturday and Laurette was sitting in a wheelchair out in the garden, where we were having a very good visit. I sat right in front of her where it was easier for her to hear what I was saying.

Laurette had not been too keen at first, but when she felt more comfortable with me she opened up and showed she still had a spark in her. Her eyes showed this side when she related how a long-ago incident in the restaurant business had not been easy on her. One day, a man threw his overdone steak at her, which was not fair as the overcooked steak was not her fault. He had stayed in the pub too long and the steak got overdone!

Laurette had worked in various professions until age seventy-two and she never tired of helping others. I asked where she was born and was surprised to hear that it was Alberta. She is a Canadian from the word go, and is proud of it. She didn't grow up on a farm but in a small French community in Alberta.

Laurette told me that early on she had wanted to be a nun as she had grown up in the Roman Catholic Church, but that she'd gotten fed up with that approach and with the church. She is still not eager about churches now.

Her parents were not rich so Laurette got her first job in her late teens. She had one sister and one brother. Her sister died at age ninety-six. Her mom died at age twenty-eight and her father died in his sixties. Her father was a carpenter. It looks like one cannot put Laurette's longevity down to heredity. Her life was poor and she learned what needs were early.

As she talked on, it was obvious that her long life had been influenced by the way she took an interest in everything that was going on around her. When she'd lived in Victoria while in her nineties, she'd instructed others how to use the computer. She liked going places, doing things, and dancing.

I took her memory way back by asking about life during the war. Had it affected her outlook on life as the years went by?

When she first came to British Columbia she lived in Vancouver, and then moved to Windsor, Ontario during the war. Her husband worked for the Ford Motor Company back then. Jim, her son, was born during the war. She doesn't think that anything back then has affected her throughout her life up to now.

When Laurette worked in a medical clinic as a medical stenographer, she told me how the doctor there had recommended that her son go into medical training as he would make a good doctor. I found out later that Jim is a retired doctor and that she thinks the world of him. This incident told me that Laurette is aware of the possibilities in other people and often thinks of how she could help them. She is wondering now what she can do at Eagle Park, the nursing home where she lives.

"How do you feel now?" I asked.

"I am always so tired," she answered. But a recent medical check-up has shown that her health is OK. "All is fine," she told me. It was an amazing answer at age a hundred and five. Her legs get very tired now though, she said, but she has always been independent.

"I look forward to the day when I die," she told me. She had known another lady in Parksville who had lived to age a hundred and eight!

It is mostly only women who live into their hundreds. "Why do so many women outlive men?" I asked her. She didn't say anything.

Now she just told me that she was tired, so I said we would finish then. But suddenly she surprised me by telling me all about how she had set up a library in the Berwick Senior Complex in Nanaimo. When she first went there, books were scattered all over the place, so she organized them into a library, and set up how everyone should use them. This looked like a good description of how Laurette looks at life. She has always tried to do something to help others, even to setting up a library system in an old folks home.

It was a real pleasure talking with Laurette. My thanks go to her friends and family for their support during her many years. She obviously has brought hope and help to many. A life well lived – all one hundred and five years.

CHAPTER 3

—

Do You Really Want To Live To 100 Years?

The more I study this possibility, the more I question my resolve. I am not sure I really want to live that long. The last thirty years have been full of pain and troubles. You are experiencing that now? So you agree? Sure we, here in Canada and the United States, are experiencing longer life on earth. What about other countries like Africa where people die in their forties? What is best for the world's people? What hopes can we cherish? What daily life is worth sharing? Now that dementia is spreading around the world, is a longer life worth hoping for? I wonder.

Obviously living in the western world where there is enough food, medicine when we are ill, and supportive communities, life goes on and on. Maybe it is better to share our food supply with poorer countries than to grab the purse for longer life. What about the men in our societies? Women outlive the men and we are not really sure why. Maybe men just do not want to live through the weaker, hurting seasons of old age. Men like to be strong and perhaps they cannot cope with the physical weakness brought on by aging. The life choice may be making a difference.

As we lose our sense of community, it may be that we are also losing our longevity. The lonely days defeat us, for it is the people you love or work with, supportive neighbours, and church friends who are there when you need them, who fill lonely days. As our society changes and the culture becomes more and more self-orientated, maybe we don't want to live into the nineties and one hundreds when we would need their help. What do you think?

If we live into our oldie years, we will want our brains to be intact. Thinking clearly and remembering those wonderful happenings of long ago is very important to aging. Your brain can give you the sense of peace and tranquility you will need as the years go by and you lose many familiar surroundings. Another very important thing to think about is how you need a positive attitude and a purpose that calls you out of yourself. Also, the more we help each other, the better we can cope through hard times. We need to maintain contact with family and friends, which is hard to do when they live so far away. When did you last learn something different to task your brain? Try learning to play the piano or learn a new language to talk with new friends, making them feel at home.

What if you were in your hundreds and had all your facilities intact? Think how wonderful it would be to still travel the world and see those spectacular sights that everyone is talking about. Try going by boat to Bermuda and discover what I mean – it is beautiful. Sure, you are in your nineties and life is truly wonderful. Or is it? Do you want to live into the hundreds?

BEPPIE'S LIFE STORY - AGE 81

How family plays an important role in the development of their "offspring," as well as circumstances for that development.

Once upon a time there was a little girl named Beppie. She lived with her parents, two sisters, and two brothers. She was born before World War II started, but she grew up in the Netherlands during the war as the country endured the occupation of German troops for five years. Amidst bombings, fear of arrest, the secret Underground, and very little food during the last two years, 1944-1945, it was a challenging time for Beppie.

Beppie's father, a businessman, had his identification falsified to make him look older, because men under forty-five had to report for duty for the Germans. Beppie's mother was a housemother; besides her own four children she also took care of ten medical students. Their five-story house was part of the local hospital. Beppie learned at a young age to help with the household chores; setting the tables, washing dishes, etc., despite the fact that they had two maids. They all worked hard. Beppie, the oldest child, had to be an example for the other children – even the neighbourhood children asked her to settle their "fights." She still feels for the underdog.

During the last years of the war, Beppie went to the communal kitchen every day with her pail and stood in long "line-ups" for seven scoops of watery soup on taste-less sauerkraut. The pail was heavy and the walk back home was long. It was a time of secrets – "Don't talk." They hid copper items, radios, and valuables under the "dumbwaiter." The radio went under the toilet where Dad and his friends, all on their bellies, listened secretly to the British Radio Broadcasting Company. It was a very stressful growing-up time. But Beppie's parents never showed any fear, and so she also felt fearless – a good quality to have.

Beppie enjoyed school, but missed two years because the school was occupied by the Germans. Eventually, after the war, children caught up but with no books, no gym, no paper, and no lab, there was just hard learning! Tenacious became the word for Beppie because she was also ill for six weeks before her final exam, and yet she did not fail. Failure is not in her vocabulary.

As children, Beppie and her siblings were raised to be methodical and neat. Family values were: loyalty to one's country and to one's family. The word obedience is not Beppie's favourite word because her parents were Calvinists and very strict.

After the war, her youngest brother, Matthew, was born in 1947. Beppie became rebellious at that time because she had not been told that her mother could have died. Her mother was very ill with toxaemia but Beppie only heard this via her neighbours. She was almost fifteen at the time. Her family was not honest with her but after her mother came home from the hospital, Beppie learned to help her care for Matthew. Beppie's words of advice are to be honest at all times with children.

A lifelong aim to help others stayed with her through-out her life – hence the nursing profession she chose. The rebellious part followed her until her "old age" and perhaps beyond still! Her dad's aggressiveness and her mom's controlling caused her grief for many years. Her mother did not show appreciation for what Beppie did — only when she was ninety-four did she tell her that she loved her. It is a lesson to tell your children, friends, or spouses that you love them.

However, Beppie sees herself as being like her mother in many ways; determined, loyal, down to earth, and a good organizer. Sensitivity and creativity were only on the back burner. Fortunately she had "surrogate" parents. Her dad's brother, a physician, took time for her and told her about the birds and the bees, music, poetry, and plays. He treated her with respect and this is what she expected from others throughout her life. Unfortunately, her uncle committed suicide, which she was told of much later. Be honest at all times!

One of the family's maids became Beppie's confidante. It is important to have someone to confide in when growing up. Beppie had lots of friends during childhood and teenage years. She could be daring and courageous at times. After high school, at the age of sixteen to seventeen, she worked in the office of a printing plant. She had to wait until she was old enough to be admitted to the school of nursing. Once she was in training, she knew she had found her purpose in life.

In 1953, after her first year in school, Beppie's parents sent her to Canada to scout for the whole family to immigrate, which was a big responsibility. She needed resilience to take care of herself in a strange country with strange customs. She spoke English! She took any job, from picking peaches in the hundred-degree weather, with heavy baskets on her shoulders, or housekeeping for two physicians in a three-story house plus an office. She learned to clean floors the hard way. All that work as a child paid off!

She married and had three children. Life was full of challenges as a new immigrant, with little money. She sewed all her own and her children's clothes. To be frugal was the word. She also had lots of fun with a local theatre group. She kept her Dutch tongue since all plays in her community then were in Dutch. During the evening, at the high school, she went to grade thirteen where she took English, biology, and chemistry, which was difficult. The prospect of getting into nursing school for the second time in her life pushed her further. Tenaciousness! In 1976, she graduated from the School of QuoVadis of Nursing, which was a two-year program for mature students. Caring for people was the right fit for her. It gave her an independent voice, appreciation, and creativity. All that she had missed in her youth she gained now.

She is thankful for all the choices she made; some good, some very bad, but she always tried not to look back and to look for new horizons.

In 1990, she sold everything in Ontario and moved to Vancouver Island, not knowing anyone. It reminded her of her immigration in 1953. This is where her fearlessness helped her to make the right decisions.

Unfortunately, her husband died after nine years of wedded bliss, but she had experienced what love can overcome. The reason to continue is to be involved – no couch potato here.

"Volunteer! Stay mentally and physically active. Thank God each day for your blessings. Look at the stars and moon and be happy!"

Beppie

CHAPTER 4

—

How Long Do I Want To Live?

Do you have to ask me that? I really don't know. I don't want to live to the place where I am a burden to family and friends. Neither do I want to lie in a bed during my last days, in a nursing home, unable to move or speak. I am in my eighties now and having trouble walking, but I can still type! So what am I going to say here? I'll be surprised if I make it to ninety, but how about you? Are you one of those people who say: I don't want to go yet – I am enjoying my life here on earth even if I am in a nursing home? There are all kinds of things I can do here, and there are many different ways I can help people. Many people are worse off than I am and I will stay as long as God gives me life.

Why are people living so long these days? Back in the 1880s people only lived to age forty, I am told. Last year, I heard from a friend of mine who was serving as a college teacher in another country that is not as well off as we are in Canada. He had noticed that his students were attending an awful lot of funerals every month or so. People were dying at forty or so in the year 2000. What is happening here that we are living so much longer now? Is it the food we eat, or the comfort we enjoy, or the medical help we receive when we are ill? Is it living more comfortably?

What am I doing to keep healthy? Do I exercise daily? Does that count towards longevity? I exercise every day in the shower – how about you? Do you at least go for a walk twice a week or so? Here in Parksville, Vancouver Island, it is lovely to go for a walk on the beach. Come and join me there some day, eh? You need the exercise and the location is absolutely beautiful.

I used to love reading books, especially murder mysteries, but now my eyes are not good and I get a headache looking too long even at the TV. What about the mind? Is it staying sharp or getting sluggish? What ways can we keep our minds sharp? How about writing a book about your life, or a story for Facebook, or staying in touch with family and friends through Social Media? That is a great idea as it will keep people in future generations sharp. But what if all that social media stuff is not your ticket for sharing – what can you do? What about the telephone, or letters? Just try, let your mind stay sharp, and active. Care about others and help others cope. I used to know a man who was bedridden, but he stayed sharp praying for others. The people in his community and church knew he would pray for their friends and families, all they had to do was ask.

For those of us who are in our nineties and who may still reach a hundred – would we want to? If we had to choose, would we choose to live that long? Surely it would depend on whether or not we were happy and healthy. We can ask God for His help too. Jesus's Spirit promises to sustain us if we ask, but would we ask? Do we still have teeth to eat with? Do we still have ears to hear the birds sing? What about moving around; do we need help all the time? Maybe real old age is too much of a disadvantage. Weakness takes its toll and we can be very weary just hanging around doing nothing. I don't think I would want to be ninety-something and be unable to function, never going out of my way to help others.

Sure we can live in our memories, but do your feelings connect now with those wonderful early years' stirring memories? I can't remember what my feelings were as I rode the bike to school along the Bermuda roads. Yes, didn't I tell you? I grew up in Bermuda but now I cannot remember the lovely scent that rose up to greet my nostrils every morning.

One good idea I have read somewhere is to limit the working hours to allow one to mature without stress. Yes, it is stress that is doing you and me in. What if your daughter only had to work four days a week instead of five, leaving time to visit you? Or what if you and your husband had taken turns working the heavy hours, leaving you each free to play with the children – less stress, right? You would probably be living longer now because of less stress. Think about it, our modern generations are suffering from stress. How can we lessen that and live happily into the future, free of the effects of stress on the body and mind? Preliminary evidence suggests that a shortened work-week may help over-extended working lives, and further increase life expectancy and better health in later years.

So friends, your old age is coming down the pike. Would you welcome it if you were strong and fit? Would you stay at home into later years offering your help to others? Will your help always be needed?

HILMER'S LIFE STORY AT AGE 90

As we sat and got comfortable, I was wondering about Hilmer's surname, Stav, which was new to me. Hilmer explained that it was Scandinavian but that his father was born in Chicago. "My parents moved there from Norway," he explained, "so we had a number of traditions meeting in my family." This is typical of Canada.

Hilmer suffers from polymyalgia rheumatica, which causes him much discomfort. It starts with pain at the back of the head and travels down the leg into the toes. "It's hard to get up early in the morning," he said. This made me think that I should set aside another chapter for people's pain and suffering in the latter years. It takes two years for this disease to really come on. "If one can get a positive view towards anything that brings on pain, one's life will be much better," Hilmer said.

Hilmer's dad settled first in the United States where he met Hilmer's mother in South Dakota, but eventually they settled in Saskatchewan in Canada where they homesteaded. His dad's job was drilling wells. Knowing the prairies, it is no wonder that back then it took forty miles, often travelling by foot, just to get to the closest store. As Hilmer remembers, it often was by horse team. However, they could order something and it would come by rail. There were eight boys and three girls in the family. Hilmer was the fifth child.

The children learned to always listen to their parents. They were all given jobs to do. Hilmer's job was to build the stove supply of kindling, even at age two. They were all organized and respected their parents who worked very hard themselves. His parent's control was positive. Discipline was based on respect for each other. Life required much of everyone. They had to walk about a mile and a quarter to school. Hilmer doesn't remember his dad talking with him, but he knows that is where he draws his strength now; from his parents and his childhood.

Hilmer wonders why he is still alive now at age ninety. His dad died at age ninety, his mother died in her eighties, and both worked very hard all day. Hilmer thinks now that because he also worked hard all his life, he should be able to get something out of this project 'sharing his story.' He appreciates this opportunity. His eagerness shows one of the gifts he has. He always looks for a new learning opportunity in everything that comes his way. Hilmer believes that if he can learn something new every day, he will not be bored with life and he is not bored with life!

As he grew older, Hilmer decided to take electricity during his senior year at school. This decision helped focus his future on his interest in the air force branch of the military. He had read a book describing WWI, which had put him off the army. His acceptance was debated as he was wearing glasses at the time so he could not fly a plane. So what could he do? Being interested in electricity led to a course on wireless mechanics in the air force.

After the war, Hilmer went back to Regina to go to school again to pick up a couple of courses he was interested in for entrance to university. Then he attended college in Regina, where veterans had their way paid. When he graduated, he applied for work. There were a hundred and fifty others applying, and he won the appointment. Afterwards, he got a job at Loon Lake as a field officer with the Department of Natural Resources. Later, he was transferred to the District of Buffalo Narrows in the northern part of Saskatchewan where he was stationed for two years. As I listened to Hilmer's story, it seemed that his job took him all over the place. At one time he had an opportunity to join his older brother in Yorkton, but sadly that did not work out.

In 1946, while in Prince Albert at Christmas time, Hilmer met the girl that was to become his wife, Margaret Lois Mitchell. Lois was training as a nurse and in 1947 they were married. As the years passed they settled in Loon Lake and had a family. They had five children but lost their first child. Lois had also been born on a farm and was a Presbyterian, so when she died in 2001, she was buried at St. Columba Presbyterian Church in Parksville, where they had been attending after retirement. They had a wonderful marriage, Hilmer says.

As the years passed, Hilmer's job took him all over. He was in charge of natural resources and later he was appointed field supervisor. He found this job very interesting. But by the time he was in his early fifties, his job put him on the go constantly, travelling to many locations. He was hardly home long enough to help with his family. Hilmer began to feel the need to have work closer to his family, which was hard to do when he was travelling around so much. He then took a little trip to Red Deer where he got a more settled job. In time, however, he realized that this wasn't what he wanted to do. Meanwhile, his wife was working as a nurse; a specialist in the hospital. Lois was a very supportive wife but Hilmer was torn and needed to make a change.

There was a job interview coming up with Consumer and Corporate Affairs. Hilmer applied and finally became a technical inspector with the federal government, in research. He worked all over Western Canada until he retired at the age of fifty-five and a half years. When I asked him about his abilities for such a job in so many places, he told me that he enjoyed the challenge and prepared himself to do the best he could. "I was my own boss," he said, and he had to be fully responsible.

In 1979, he and Lois came to Vancouver Island as his daughter lived in Campbell River. Interested in moving there, they could see all the positive things about living on the Island. After talking it over, they felt there was tremendous potential there. They started looking for a three-bedroom house. There was a house for sale in Qualicum Beach that interested them, and they got it for a good price. "It was truly a gift," he said. They moved here to Vancouver Island in October of 1979.

As Hilmer's story wound down I asked him, "Of what in your life are you most proud? Where did you learn to evaluate a situation so thoroughly before you moved into it?"

He thought for a minute then said, "As you go through life, you meet so many who are just jumping in here and there and are sorry afterwards. I adapted well with my eyes wide open. I just tried to stay within my limits. I also had a good marriage. Lois was a wonderful person and she provided help if she could.

"Where I grew up there was no talk of God," Hilmer said. "It was a long walk to church. The neighbour was Roman Catholic and she walked to her church. I never had a private conversation with my dad about anything. My mom had more connections with God and church originally. Our family connection was that of respect. My inner soul guiding me was strong; fashioned in my childhood. I hate to think about children today growing old.

Where is the respect that will get them through life? They are all adrift, having no connection with the community around them."

"How do you manage the pain in your body as it grows weaker?" I asked Hilmer.

His answer: "I asked medical people what to do about the pain, but my doctor just looked far away and said very little. I wonder now if I should take Aleve for pain. I just keep going as well as I can. I have learned to manage many experiences and jobs in my life, and now it is me I have to manage. I have had a hard time giving up driving," Hilmer admitted. "I was looking forward to getting a scooter and today I just learned there is one coming. Sure I have difficulty getting out and about, but for years I have loved going down to the beach, watching people, especially children playing, and striking up conversations with people. Now I am real excited to be able to do it again with the scooter. I understand it is red so people can be aware of me as I go by enjoying my scooter!

"Yes, I have had a lot of time to ponder my life and see the bigger picture. I am not optimistic about the future. I have to keep careful tabs on my medications, and that is not easy as my short-term memory is not good. My family gathered for my ninetieth birthday a few days ago, which uplifted my spirits especially. While talking with my last remaining brother about 'old times,' which had all been stirred by this job now, recalling my memories way back to childhood, I wonder about it all.

"I've been thinking and want to say this: As we get older we have time to sort things out, basically, so one can feel comfortable – our lives fulfilled to the best of our abilities. But we, as elders, and I admit it, have taught our siblings many things over the years. Unfortunately, depending on their circumstances, we have taught our kids to be responsible, but they forget about the needs of their senior relatives who had helped them so much in the early years. Sadly, they still do not do what we would like them to do. We phone and they don't come, not even from my own family. I am left now on my own but it was my daughter living in Alberta who arranged for my scooter!"

I asked Hilmer if he could share with me where his personal confidence came from. He said, "I learned to do what my parents asked me to do. We all struggled. We all had to share, learning how to take responsibility from within and for the family. The youngest in our family took his own life. That was hard. Yet today, the more we get the less we respect. We were a big family and we all had to put a positive effort into things. If you were given a job you had to do it! I worry today about my grandchildren. Their lives today are too easy."

After he had shared all this, I thanked Hilmer for being open and honest with me. We had a great visit and I really appreciated Hilmer's willingness to lay his life's journey out for me.

CHAPTER 5

—

The Spark That Extends Human Life

Everywhere I visited with aging oldies I asked the same question, "What is the spark that has lengthened your life into the nineties or one hundreds?" It is a great question, right? Everyone had a different reply. Some have told me that they always find everything interesting. Others have said that they are intrigued with each day's possibilities. Another response was, "I intend to live forever. It is so far, so good." If you are in your nineties as you read this book, what would you say?

Much research has been done on the health of the aged population. One writer suggests the aging population should put their attention on making friends. I like that, for loneliness does make us sorrowful and tired. It's not a good acceptance of self. Surely self-acceptance has something to do with successful aging into the nineties and one hundreds.

What other factors are good clues to healthy aging in any decade? Depression or self-pity will not be one of them. Is there a certain self-perspective among them? What about keeping busy and active? Surely that has something to do with life's longevity. Just sitting around in a chair will not do it. How about self-sacrifice? How much does one give to another, in love, in friendship, to fill another's needs, or in support, even when one is also hurting? How much does one give self away in order to live longer? Is this the basis of happiness? Could this be the basis of longevity? I am writing this book at age eighty-two – will this effort give me longer years to be active and interested in life itself?

How one deals with stress, in both personal and family situations, may also lengthen life. How often have we taken something to relax us when worried stiff about a loved one? Would worry upset one's life span or does it depend on how we deal with those worries? I commit them to God. Other friends talk them over with others and they do not get blown away by their weight. By the way, does weight itself have anything to do with life's longevity? Probably, but I am not a physician. I only know that when my weight gets beyond a hundred and sixty pounds I feel old and unattractive.

When you read Monica's life story, you will notice that she lives in the present day, regardless of her health. She says to me, "I intend to live forever," and she means it, regardless of how she feels. This means she is positive about each day. I suggest to you, my readers, that staying healthy and having a positive view of life are both from the same thought progression. Along with not smoking, which is a huge no-no, and having good genes, what else can we actually do to achieve long life? Sure, one's health will affect it, but what about one's attitude towards self and others?

A spiritual awareness of human potential suggests to us that what will really count as the years go by is love; the God-given love that is based on unselfishness. Do you and I put others first – put their needs before our own? That takes much thought. Even when one is involved in a happy marriage, one or the other usually comes first. Perhaps you've been involved in an accident. Do you think of the others that are hurt before your own needs? What extends life; giving it away, or holding on for dear life?

When we feel positive about our lives, this also extends our inner souls as we go through each day. We gain self-respect and self-acceptance. This means that we are not pulling ourselves apart. The lack of self-acceptance may truly lead to an early death. We do not even like ourselves so why should we put up with this tomfoolery any more? I am so tired of self. I am leaving. I die.

One thing a Christian has that extends life way into the future is the joy of living. As long as we hold on to God's gift, that wonderful view of self that brings joy and gladness, life will go on and on. One may even reach a hundred, living a life of joy. At least that is what I have heard when talking with people in their nineties and one hundreds. I've appreciated talking with all of them very much. It has been a privilege.

MONICA'S LIFE STORY AT AGE 95

"My name is Monica and I am ninety-five years old. There is a question as to what to call me. My second name is Monica and my first name is Mary. At my birth, the extended family had five girls who were all called Mary because they wanted to honour Mary. However, everyone knows me as Monica now, which is my second name so that is what I am called in this, my life story. I start by saying: So far, so good! Yes, I intend to live forever. The devil does not want me and I cannot get to Heaven on my own, so here I am."

This opening statement shows Monica's spirit: come what may, I am here to stay. Monica enjoys life and takes an interest in it, and in dogs especially. Her dog was the first to meet me at the door.

Monica, however, wants to begin her story from her childhood years. She wants to pay close attention to the differences between the early 1900s and today. The gaps are immense, especially in the lives of girls. Monica was brought up in the post-Victorian Era; born in 1919 in Winnipeg where the family lived comfortably in a large house. Both of her parents were music teachers. Her father was a violinist and her mother also taught music. There were five pianos and two studios in the house. Monica learned the cello and piano. Her dad was a strict teacher and rather hard on his girl. Girls had no standing back then and were not expected to develop into anything much, even though Monica's mother had graduated from the Royal Academy of Music.

Monica's parents were originally from England and well off, but somehow Monica had not gained an appreciation of herself. Her dad ignored her most of the time and the family did not help her gain any self-respect. She went to a Catholic school but when she was around age fourteen to seventeen years old, the Depression period in 1930 hit the family very hard, so they went back to England as her brother had received a music scholarship there.

As she looked back on her childhood, I asked Monica to describe her personal feelings. She admitted that she had been really timid for many years – after all, her brother got all the attention, right? She remembers how her brother got a toy tank one year while she got one much smaller. That demonstrates how she was seen in the family – small and insignificant.

Monica was a quiet, obedient, little girl who felt rather anxious all the time. Was this true all her life? She attended the Roman Catholic Church where she was filled with anxiety, for you went to Hell if you didn't obey and go to church. Not being a boy made her very anxious about herself and that anxiety, she admits, is still in her. Her personality was socially timid; wanting to get along but not wanting to rub people the wrong way. Looking back, she remembers how her father started to teach her to play the violin. She recalls asking him, "Why can I not play big notes like you?" He just laughed at her then and she still feels dismissed and laughed at and not really cared for by her dad. He never tried to teach her anything after that happened, so she dropped the violin and switched to her mother's piano lessons.

I asked Monica: what were her gifts now? Immediately it came out strong, "I am very social. I like people. I wanted to play with my friends as a teenager, but was forced to practice after school. I never had much time to play." So Monica turned to dogs all her life. Dogs loved her and they gave her a chance to be social. She still has one. Monica made a good life out of training, showing, and breeding dogs.

When Monica married Roy, he was a music student who was taking lessons from her father. Roy was also a Presbyterian and not Roman Catholic, so her parents didn't approve of the marriage. However, it was a good marriage for sixty-two years. Roy was protective and cared for her, which was a new experience for Monica. They produced two girls and a boy, and Monica finally learned what it was like to be accepted for herself. In her childhood family, the maids, cooks, and everyone who served the family home looked after all of them well, but did not show the children that they were appreciated. Monica had stopped school after grade ten and later had learned to be a secretary. Few jobs were open to teenage girls back then.

Now married, Monica was accepted and finally happy. Looking at her, I asked, "What challenged you to grow to be the woman you are today, confident and sure of yourself?" It was the dogs, she said. Surprised, I asked her to describe what she meant. How could dogs change her whole attitude towards herself?

Monica explained, "I was totally dedicated to animals, especially dogs." She worked for many years with dogs and they gave her confidence. Monica bred dogs, gave obedience training classes, and received love and respect from the dogs and their handlers. Enjoying the confidence and position of authority, she developed a way to respond to people and to feel confident about her inner self. Her confidence grew from the love of dogs and what they drew from her. She later expanded her interest to training tracking dogs and she did not quit until she was seventy-five. It was the community of dog people that gave Monica self-respect, and she had a specific place in it. "I had come into my own," she said.

I asked Monica, "What was the spark in your life that has made you accept life as given to you now?"

Her answer didn't surprise me. "The spark in my life was the dogs and the way I connected with life," she said. "I am interested in being alive! My general health is good, the doctor says."

Yes, it is obvious she is enjoying life and taking an interest in it and in dogs especially.

When they first retired, Monica and Roy stayed several days in Vancouver where they spent Christmas with four friends. Then they came as visitors to Parksville. She had never felt so at home before, but now she did. Other places were always demanding attention, but here it felt so peaceful. So Monica moved to Parksville, Vancouver Island from Winnipeg in her seventies and she loved it. After Winnipeg's winters, the weather on the Island was superb. The children were now adults living their own lives. There was just her and Roy and they travelled all over the Island, enjoying life. Retirement was good! Sure there were allergies to mosquito bites, but nothing much really hurt. They had come with one dog but now they bought two more Golden Retrievers.

Life was good. The people living in their community were really friendly. The ambiance itself was friendly and Monica had confidence in their new home. They were in the right place; a good neighbourhood – home. "I never felt at home on the prairies," she said. "In your seventies you must look forward, not backward. I reinvented myself. People got to know the real me. Here was a new opportunity." She had shaken off the shadows of Winnipeg. "Bad memories I tried to leave behind," she told me. "Here was a new opportunity. People are so friendly – they accept you. The climate itself was open."

When Roy died in 2002, Monica was eighty-two years old but you never would have guessed it. Alone now, she continued to enjoy each day as it came, and continued with her friends. Monica never complained of being lonely. She just enjoyed her life and welcomed each day as it came. Together with her two dogs she lived confidently alone. Finally, many years later, she welcomed her daughter who had come to live with her.

"What was the spark that kept you going?" I asked Monica.

"I have always done what I thought was right at the time," she said. "I did my best and I always tried. I thank God that I have been so fortunate, having escaped the turmoil in the world. I had no cancer and I still have my wits about me. I am thankful every day for the day itself. I have some back pain but it's not constant. I thank God for the fortunate life I have had. I had postpartum depression when the kids were born, but I did not let it defeat me. I could wake up and enjoy the world and I did! God gave me an inner peace. I had done the best I could. Nothing was perfect but I did my best. I have never dealt with people out of malice. If I am not interested I just walk away. I don't go looking for traits I do not like. I just go the other way. I try to keep myself on an even keel."

At ninety-five, Monica reflects, "I look back at my life now and see the positive side not the negative. I can see the faults but I don't dwell on them. My life is like a painting. I don't dwell on the brush strokes, but on the total picture of who I am now. This is me."

CHAPTER 6

—

How Can We Cope?

As I talk with people in their older years; the eighties, nineties, and one hundreds, I can't fail to notice that everywhere there is despair. Older seniors are confined to beds or to chairs at home, or their home is now in a nursing residence under supervision. How can we cope if we lose our independence? When I look around, most are women sitting there, looking sadly at me. I wonder about the future God has planned for me.

When I visit the Eagle Park Nursing Home, most of the patients are women. Women also are more anxious to talk with me than men. They want to tell me their stories, but men are more reluctant. They are not anxious to talk. They know only too well that their daily lives have been based on their personal ability to cope on their own. Why is this? During the older years have we lost the means to live adequately on our own? Is this why we are so down?

What about the men? Have men also lost their way, having lost their ability to be self-reliant? Is this true of all of us in our future years? When I visited with Hilmer who is age ninety, I learned that sadly, his wife died years ago leaving him alone. Now he is stuck at home, unable to drive, unable to have any manner of movement outside, other than walking or being driven by a friend. Even his meals are delivered. Can you feel his sense of loss?

But this is also the situation with older women who live alone at home, as they slowly move into the nineties and become unable to cope on their own. This is not a separate issue with men and women. It is true of anyone aging as they are having difficulty managing on their own. Stuck inside, unable to function as they used to, they are slowly going through the nineties feeling bereft. Will such sadness mean that we don't wish to live into the one hundreds? Would you want to live beyond where you are now, where you can be efficient and helpful to others, beyond where you can look after yourself? No? I don't blame you.

I sometimes wonder if God meant any of us to live beyond where we could help another, spreading His love in the action. Let us pray about it as we read this chapter and book. Let us not let the sadness close our minds to what is possible. Maybe you will see something as you read on that will help you make the situation more bearable, where love can be shared effectively as we help one another.

MY OWN LIFE STORY AT AGE 82

I was born in Windsor, Nova Scotia and am thankful to be a Canadian, but when I was four months old, the family moved to Hamilton, Bermuda where Dad was the Presbyterian minister at St. Andrews. I loved growing up in Bermuda, but as the middle child with an older sister and younger brother, I didn't get much attention from my parents and grew up shy and neglected. My brother says we grew up in a fragmented family. Dad spent most of his time fulfilling the needs of church members, and mother felt my brother could do no wrong. When my sister returned after a year away at college, I saw Dad give her a big hug. I was in the dining room and I can see them still in the kitchen. I wondered why he wouldn't give me such a hug. He never did – only a whipping a few times, when I admit I probably deserved it.

Back then, in the 1940s, the world was just recovering from the Second World War. When I look back at days spent in the Bermuda High School for Girls, I recall that I had few friends and often was left standing under a tree all by myself. My dad, being a minister, was also on the School Governing Board – a scary relationship to be ignored. I felt neglected but I passed each Form as they were called; it being the English system. The rare time I was recognised was on sports day when I ran races and always won, unless there were any girls of colour in the line-up. They always outran me.

When it was my turn to come to Canada to get an education, I chose to attend the Toronto School of Music for a piano degree. I was going to be a concert pianist but God had other ideas. Even though I was neglected often at home, I now came into my own. I was staying at the Deaconess School, open just to girls, so I felt right at home. A year later I decided to go into the Deaconess Training Program and when I graduated I started working in several churches. Unfortunately, they really only wanted a church secretary, not a deaconess. I was not appreciated, so when I finally left I returned home to discover what a deaconess could do in Bermuda and had a great year. Mother had died in the meantime and Dad needed some help. When he got married again, I played the wedding march as they left the church, which was a strange feeling. Returning to Canada and having finished my degree, I went into the Peace area of Alberta and British Columbia where the churches were very undermanned. But a woman? They loved me and I finally found myself.

I decided to return to college, so went to Winnipeg where I took Bachelor of Arts courses to prepare me to attend Knox College. The Presbyterian Church had finally ordained women. While in Winnipeg, I started an after-school program in my home, which drew in many children and teenagers. It was the start of Flora House, an inner city mission that has lasted to this day. This was around 1967.

Later, while in Alberta, I started a church in a hall in Red Deer. As a deaconess, I couldn't baptise any babies or children so my dad came out from British Columbia and baptised many babies for me. He enjoyed it and was finally loving and accepting me as a deaconess. It was a special service.

After graduation from Knox College, I was finally ordained. I was the twentieth woman to be ordained in the Presbyterian Church. Everywhere I went, though, they had never known a woman minister. One man came to hear me give the Call to Worship and decided to stay for I was not that bad. It was hard on me though, never knowing if I would be accepted. Later I became the Moderator of that Presbytery. I was the first woman in more than a hundred years to be elected Moderator of the

Presbytery, and only the third in Canada to gain such a position. I was getting used to being partially accepted but never really. Maybe it was in my own brain I was not good enough. I built that church up to a sizable congregation and the building was erected. We were a family church there in Waterloo, but when I left, the male minister that followed me tried to return the church to male dominance. The small family groups I had started were no more.

Through all this rigmarole, I went out west to British Columbia where I was asked to take on another new congregation, which I did. This congregation also grew and grew, finally meeting in their own mobile structures, which were shared with the Koreans. But when I finally retired, everything went wrong and the families that had enjoyed the puppet shows I had put on of Bible stories stopped attending, as did their children. Now, without the family emphasis, most churches only have seniors attending or have closed.

Meanwhile, over the years, with the ups and downs of church work, I was writing books, and have nine published in all. One was called *Coming Alive Together*, and dealt with small groups in churches. Another was called *Spiritual Muffins* and was about spiritual food, which I felt many were lacking as the church continued to decline. The last one, written after retirement, was called *My Life's Labyrinth* and described the faith journey as we walk with Jesus through life.

I moved with a friend to Sechelt on the Sunshine Coast, and together we bought a recreational vehicle and travelled the United States, Mexico, and Canada enjoying ourselves. Yes, I was finally enjoying myself and had a good friend who accepted me as I was; not a perfect minister at all. Finally we moved to Vancouver Island where I am writing this life story. Dorothy has now died and I am on my own again, but my way ahead is clear. The real service in the ministry of God is how we love others and serve them faithfully as God directs us. I think I was on the right track years ago when I worked with families, thanks to the deaconess training. God gave me a good foundation that served me well through my years as I faithfully served Him and wrote the book *Coming Alive Together*.

These days, I am attending St. Columba Church where I now worship. I look back with gratitude. God has brought me through many wrinkles. When I was first here, I wrote and put on an annual Christmas Play that was enjoyed by the families and individuals in them. Now as I age, I wonder. Not all I did was perfect but in His love people loved and accepted me as a minister of His Church, and faithfully we came together to church week after week and loved one another. Yes, ministry is just that, leading all of us through the years by the grace of God, in and through a church fellowship. This is what being a church is all about – a community enjoying God's love as we share worship together and serve others in His love. I finally learned what real love is all about. I no longer feel left out. I belong to God's family.

CHAPTER 7

—

Dealing With Aches And Pains

Oh the aching! How can I move and get out of bed in the morning when I am so sore? Everyone I speak to in my age range is the same way. At first I was blaming it on the coming fall and winter, for as the weather changes, the cold winds blow, and rain descends I ache more and more. What really does cause it? Sure arthritis must be the culprit but what to do about it? Several years ago, a truck hit me and broke my right shoulder in three places. Now my shoulders hurt as well as my hips and feet. Darn! See, it isn't just aging but aging sure brings out the worst as the years go on and on.

If it is arthritis that is bothering you and me, it can progress until it affects one's ability to move in every direction. How long can you stand on your feet without a walking stick? Perhaps you are already looking at walkers and judging their effectiveness for you. I have been looking at them but wonder what leaning into the walker will do to my shoulders. Life is so different than just a few years ago when I was an athlete, playing tennis, golf, and swimming etc. Swimming was my usual activity in the summer and fall but now look at me. Darn! Aging is no fun, right? Well, don't let it get you down, for depression and that sad feeling of loss does not help one move around. What does your health professional say about it?

How do we live with pain? I have been told that a good diet with lots of fruit and vegetables helps ease the pain for it maintains a healthy weight so you are not dragging a bigger body around. Yet, there is a purpose in the pain, for God does not allow us to suffer needlessly. What have you and I learned so far? Patience! Ease of mind without needless worry when there isn't anything we can do to change the big picture. But pain isn't just something to be tolerated. What can we learn in this season of our lives? What can we learn from the pain? If pain is a normal part of aging then think again. Sure, it is always prevalent, but is life trying to show us something we need to learn? How best to walk, for instance? How best to sleep? How best to get through each day without complaining? Can we just blot it out of our minds and go on living happily ever after? I have been told firmly that arthritis is not a normal part of aging, but it sure can seriously diminish quality of life. Its presence means there is a lot of inflammation of a joint or joints. Osteoarthritis is there from the wear and tear on the cartilage and joints. Cartilage cushions the bones at the joints and when it breaks down and wears away, the bones rub together causing pain, swelling and stiffness. I can feel it happening in me as I write. Pain! Those darn joints become less flexible and stiff. The cartilage begins to rub together. Even the finger joints change. I don't like the sound of that as I love to play the piano and organ.

What can we do to ease the pain and stiffness? Get moving and watch your weight. Exercise every day to strengthen your muscles. I take a shower every day and do an exercise routine with the hot water flowing from the shower over my sore muscles. Be careful though, do not slip and fall. Make sure you have safety grips on each side of the shower. Bones do become more brittle as we age and may break more easily. I know someone who has been through several surgeries because she fell and broke her back in the tub.

Last thought is to take a well-balanced meal with adequate amounts of calcium and keep a cheery face so you can encourage others, for we are all aging together.

LIFE STORY OF ELAINE AT AGE 84

"I wanted to call my life dull, but as I shared my story I could see that dull was not right. My life was good and stable. I was born in Exeter, Ontario in 1930 to Elva and Thomas. I was their adored only child. My dad was an auto mechanic working on cars in their early days. My mom played the piano and was a stay-at-home mom who also took in boarders. Exeter was a very small town. Our home was a two-story structure with electricity, where we had a very comfortable life. When I was five years old I went to grade one at school. There it was all routine, yes, stable as my parents were well settled.

"At age fifteen I was a waitress at Grand Bend Summer Resort. Later, I worked at a restaurant in London, Ontario during the Christmas holidays. A man called William popped in one day as he was on leave from the Air Force. His station was at St. Thomas. We absolutely clicked. I was just sixteen then, but he kept coming back as he liked the look of me and we finally got married. My parents had no choice as I had made up my mind. That is what girls did back then – they got married. No one pushed me in school or later either. My husband had the same interests as my dad but he travelled around quite a bit. We moved first to London, Ontario then finally on to British Columbia where his dad had a gas station at the Lake of the Woods location. My husband was quite like my dad, who I really loved from childhood on as he was an angel of a man. We had a good marriage with three children; a girl and two boys. My daughter Paula lives in Prince George and is my rock these days as she comes whenever I call her. Bradley went to university and has a steady job at MacMillan Bloedel. Martin is a school teacher in Alberta. Paula has six grandchildren.

"Every summer we travelled a great deal, taking long drives in our car. We also moved our home from place to place a lot, as my husband had a restless streak, always looking for something better. We settled in Goderidge, Ontario, and also kept going back to Exeter several times as my parents were still there. We also went to British Columbia where Bill's parents lived. Bill was always looking for 'greener pastures' as he had lots of get up and go.

"When we finally settled in Prince George, British Columbia, I was a telephone operator at B.C Tel for eighteen years and worked in the office. We bought a house and settled down to raise a family, and our kids grew up there in British Columbia. Unfortunately, Bill developed health problems. He was a big man but diabetes cut down his strength. Finally his heart gave out and sadly he died.

We were married from 1947 to 2005. I loved him and miss him now.

"My daughter Paula has been a nurse in Kamloops and she has given me four grandchildren. Bradley, my second son, is an accountant, a good lad, and he has given me one granddaughter. My third son, Martin, is a schoolteacher in Alberta, and he has two girls. Paula has six grandchildren – two live in England. I have six great-grandchildren. Paula learned stability from me, I guess, as she is a very stable person. She did not get it from my husband. I was dull but he was exciting! Now in my eighties one forgets the bad stuff and just remembers the good.

"In my early years I went to church as my mother was a Protestant. My husband, though, was not interested so we drifted away. However, I was always the security for our family. We kept going back to Exeter in Ontario where my parents still lived, as we needed support at times.

"Four years ago, my daughter met an interesting man downtown. She invited him over to my place as he was really nice. He is ninety-three years old so he is older than me. We are company for each other. I don't know what I'd do without Harry. It would be terribly lonely.

"I forgot to tell you that we ran a pet shop in Prince George called 'PET S n THINGS' for many years. We had dogs and cats all the time at home and in our store there were the usual animals: parrots, canaries, budgies, guinea pigs etc. We also had a miniature horse we called Charlie, who lived in our backyard in Suburbia.

"One thing that I have trouble thinking back on was when I was suffering from cancer several years ago. I have probably blotted it out of my mind because it is too painful to think about. Today I have a good doctor's health assessment and I am so thankful.

"That is my entire story I can remember. You wonder about my life now? I am just drifting along. Happy in my own little world, not bored at all, just content. Yes, that's a good description of my life now in my eighties – just content. What is exciting in old age? As seniors, we put a lot right out of our minds as it is too painful now to think about. I carry on as best as I can. I tend to look at my whole life as stable even when my husband had us drifting along. Home life was a challenge but I always felt safe and secure. You go with the flow. I am just naturally stable. My grandchildren, in their hectic lives today, don't come by here often but I suspect they look on my life as stable compared to theirs. Today they don't actually look in on me. That is why I wonder if they see me as dull. Has my life been dull? I wouldn't say so. Stable is a better word."

CHAPTER 8

—

A Plan For Your Life

Have you ever wondered how things were put together to make a life? What if God had a plan for your life? Would that make it any easier when you are trying to make a decision that won't come easy? What if God had already put your life together even before you were born? That's crazy Iris, you would say. But as you look back now over your life, there were many different ways it came together, all the way to this eightieth year. Do you think there was any control over your events? What about your engagement? Did God have that all worked out before you put the question?

Scripture says rather definitely that God knows what is needed in your life and when you ask for His leading, things come together in amazing ways. A verse that has always helped me is, "I trust in you, Lord. I say. You are my God. My times are in your hands." Psalm 31:14. How about this one? "With long life I will satisfy them and show them my salvation." God knows where we are as oldies. Our times are in His hands. You don't have to feel lonely, or downcast. Look up! Plans are being made right now for your blessing. They will bring things together for you in amazing ways.

When you finish reading the story that Hazel and David share here, you too will be asking, "Was there any plan in place over my life, or was it just me making decisions, or Dad showing the way?" Are you a believer in a Divine Plan? Think about all the mistakes you have made or the direction your path took that brought you to a place you never dreamed of. The question is a far-reaching one: Am I fully responsible for my life, or am I following a greater plan Divinely put together? Do I matter to God that much? Wow!

ALL THE WAY
HAZEL'S LIFE STORY AT AGE 87

"My early days were in Saskatchewan where the family had a farm quite a distance from town and even farther from a city. I had one brother who has since died. My mom played the violin and my most meaningful memory of her was when she was playing, which she did often for hymn sings and church meetings. Most church services back then were in a home somewhere on the prairies, often in ours, and the local people conducted them. I can remember once my dad made up five gallons of ice cream as a treat for the people who came. The violin tune that flows through my head is, "All the Way my Saviour Leads Me." Its message has seen me through all my life.

"When I was in my teens, the family moved to Manitoba to a much larger house. There was a church and our house became a bunk-down place for clergy visiting to take the services. It also became the church meeting place for lots of activities like Bible studies. Through it all, Mom always sat with me for bedtime prayers. She was also involved with the Women's Missionary Society. I remember once coming home to get a special dress, only to discover that it had been put in a box and shipped off to a little Indian girl.

"In high school, I worked as a switchboard operator in the Telephone Office on weekends as money was scarce. This was the Depression years. I needed to save money to go to college. I answered phone calls at night, changed into good clothes in the morning, and then went and preached somewhere. Ministers were scarce back then but God was moulding me for my future. Finally it was time to go to college. I remember taking off for Brandon College by bus. There were no cars in our family. I met my future husband David there at college. It was God's leading.

"Too young and inexperienced you think. Regular prayers were the norm for this home. God was leading me. I was on my way to a life of service in the church and Presbytery had many little, vacant churches waiting for me. That was life on the prairies in the forties. I felt called to a life of service for God in His Church, but being a woman, how could I fit in? I finally attended the Presbyterian Mission and Deaconess Training School for women where I graduated in 1952. I remember how one of the other girls there, a Val Ford (Iris's sister) put a stuffed alligator in my bed. Women were not in clergy positions then, the Deaconess School was my only opening to further my studies. I found, however, that much of the studies there were just repeated learning from my college days and I was bored at first. I finally majored in Theological and Christian Education studies and also did some studies in the Chinese Language at the University of Toronto.

"In 1952, I was designated as a deaconess in Hartney, Manitoba. David had an opportunity to meet my parents back then. He tells the story this way: 'One winter Sunday when I was going to supply St. Paul's Church in Hartney, and knowing I would be lunching with the Turnbulls (Hazel's parents) I invited their daughter Hazel, (whom I had met in one of my classes) to go with me. She agreed, but as we were turning off the main road into town there was a blowing snow storm and the car slipped off the road. I had to walk and get help from a farm and of course was late for the service, but was welcomed by the few who had turned out. Hazel was just someone who I had met and who had left Brandon to go east to further college training and wasn't heard from again by me. Little did I know then what God was leading me into.'"

Hazel continues, "My oldest daughter will eventually get the special Bible I received at my designation and hopefully she will keep it in a special place. Afterwards, I was expected to take Summer Mission Appointments for the work experience, conducting daily vacation Bible Schools, camps etc. in Saskatchewan and Manitoba, my home turf. I longed to have a violin and Mom's violin still echoes in my ear – "All the way my saviour leads me," and the Lord's leading has led me all the way.

"My first appointment with the Board of Missions (or Women's Missionary Society) was to teach grades one and two at Cecilia Jeffrey School in Kenora, Ontario. I was there for two years and will never forget rocking the children to sleep as they cried. They were native children forcibly taken from their homes. It was a sad two years there for me.

"My next appointment was to the Chinese Presbyterian Church in Montreal where I did the same kinds of things as I had done in Toronto. The Mission Board also involved me in doing Extension Work in Yorkton, Saskatchewan and in West Toronto where new congregations were springing up and churches were being started.

"Then the Lord had other plans for me. I had already met David in Brandon College when we were both students. After several years we reconnected when David arrived in Toronto for Theological Studies at Knox College.

"Looking back, the Lord has led me to serve Him in many ways: on camp committees, the Canadian Girls In Training Board, and Girls Work secretary. I've been a church school teacher, and member of two ladies groups. Also, I've served as a representative elder in Saanich Peninsula and Chair of the Synod's Church Growth Committee. Recently I've retired as Women's Missionary Society President but still hear God's message echoing in my heart from my mother's violin years ago – all the way my Saviour is leading me.

CHAPTER 9

—

Sharing Aging

"Grow old with me! The best is yet to be."
— *Robert Browning*

It is a pleasure to talk with those who have aged together and shared long life for many, many years. God created Adam and brought Eve into the picture, giving them happiness as they toiled together on this earth. Couples today, however, tend to put off until a later year building family life. The job and security is more important these days. Money is what makes the basis of a family life. Is this really the way it should be?

When we look at couples who have aged together, there is a sharing of life together that draws the best out of each. They share the spark that enables them to live a happy life for many years. It is even more special when the spark is shared between them and all through the lives of their children. It shows in what the children accomplish in their lives. They really live and contribute something wonderful to the earth. It is a continuation of the family's spark.

Robert Browning is in my family tree I am told, and from him I have gained this writing gift. Unfortunately, so many oldies have the worry of ill health to contend with, making it difficult for them to adventure into new avenues of promise. However, God will see us all through as the months and years go by and God's love strengthens us. We are supported by each other's love as our two friends are, who share their story here.

The Scripture that has kept our two friends together for so many years shows in their life stories given here. It is Proverbs 3:6. "In all your ways acknowledge Him, and He shall direct your paths."

CONTINUING ALL THE WAY
DAVID'S LIFE STORY AT AGE 86

"I have many early memories of a very happy childhood home where prayer, grace at meals, and church attendance were all very important. But from what I have heard, I must have been very curious as a boy, following the bread cart down the street, leaving my mother to find me. Once when she was going out, and my brother was out too, Mom tied me to the clothesline where I could run up and down and even play in my sand box while still tied. I don't remember much from those years when I was just four or five years old. I must have worried my parents at times but I knew I was loved.

"In our home church, there were two services every Sunday. This was a community of working folk on the north side of Regina, Saskatchewan. God was always there and I also went to Sunday school. When I was in my teens, the Sunday school superintendent encouraged me to think of ministry as a career. How could this be possible in the Depression? Eventually the Session, the Church governing body, asked me to help in a developing area in Moose Jaw. Also, in my last year in high school I was hired by T. Eaton Company to work in men's wear on Saturdays.

"God had plans ahead of me and I can see that now. Our former minister from Regina, now in Brandon, encouraged me to go to college in Brandon and take arts. He was encouraging me to prepare for the ministry. Even then, God was planning ahead for this fellow from a working family – me. I didn't have much money to go on, so I babysat this minister's son while both his parents worked. I also received board and room in this working arrangement. While there, I received a call from T. Eaton's

Company. They had heard I was there and could I give them another half-day? I did!

"God was obviously working in mysterious ways. The minister, in whose home I was boarding, finally moved to Ontario. The Presbytery and Interim Moderator asked if I would take on supplying the pulpit on Sundays. This meant I had to move out of the manse, to where? Then a lady from the congregation and her grandson offered me free room and board as part of their offering to God. Wow! When the church finally called a minister, one of the other churches became vacant and so I continued Sunday supply. I also supplied in other churches nearby, one being Hartney. There I met the Turnbull family, Hazel's family, as they always fed and housed the Sunday supply that came to their little church.

"When I finally left for Knox College in Toronto, I had never been that far from home but God had a plan. My years at Knox were very faith-filling and busy. I sang in the Knox College Choir, and when we went on tour I was chosen as the choir student manager. The tour took us from Kitchener, Ontario to Victoria, British Columbia and back to Toronto through the northern United States. We visited high schools and sang songs on the radio. We also sang in local churches and were fed by congregations. We travelled by bus, 'The Golden Chariot' we called it, from one of our favourite songs, and we were in a bus painted gold. This was a preaching-singing mission.

"While studying at Knox, the students were appointed by the Board of Missions to small, rural churches to conduct vacation Bible schools and to preach on Sundays. I learned a lot from doing whatever pastoral work was needed. I remember one particular appointment being given keys to an old car that had to be parked on an incline, keys in the ignition, and the brake off − give it a push and then it would start. It eventually gave out and I was given a bike to ride to various points in the charge. I would often be given a drink of milk supplied by several families along the way. When all this became too much, I was supplied with a horse. These are great memories. God continued His plan for my life − a young man, certain of His call to Ministry from a very ordinary Christian family − Depression-born, from a working class home, but God continued His plan.

"During my last year at Knox, I was asked to go to Ottawa on weekends to work under the Extension Committee. This required going by train Friday night or Saturday a.m., and back overnight on Sunday for Monday classes. Boy, they kept me moving and as a result, instead of this Western fellow going back to the West upon graduation, I was appointed to the Ottawa Presbytery as, "Extension Missioner." I was to assist in developing four new congregations, which were meeting in schools on a Sunday. Three years after completing my studies at Knox College, Hazel and I were married. It was the start of many years of married bliss as we were and are very happy together.

"By this time, what with working in new extension churches, I also helped with workshops in western Canada. One of the congregations was West Point Grey in Vancouver and they eventually called me as their minister. Years later, God was still planning ahead for our lives. I was called to Knox Church, Victoria in 1976 to a growing congregation. The sanctuary was increased in size while I was there. An addition was built to contain a church hall, kitchen, lounge and vestry, library, and nursery. In many ways I was still doing extension work with the building and congregation.

"In 1983, God saw me through bypass heart surgery. We were blessed to have five retired clergy and two deaconesses in the congregation who helped see us through this. Because of heart issues continuing off and on, I retired in 1989.

"God continues to amaze Hazel and me, working in mysterious ways, planning ahead of us, leading us on. Several of our family members are involved in the life and work of the church where they live. One grandson is a youth pastor, and another is instrumental in a church planted on the Mainland. While thinking of our kids, over the years Hazel reminds me of the Sunday when our son, who we had in church that day, disappeared. After calling the police, they found him finally asleep in the pulpit. I wonder what God will make of that eventually. Another story she tells is of a very young neighbour boy who watched her washing one day when she had a black cleric shirt in the sink. He wondered why she waited so long to wash it until it got that black.

"As I look back, I realise that if Hazel had not had deaconess training it would have been hard for her. She encouraged me so much. Life together was never a problem as we talked over everything in the family and prayed about it. Looking back now I can see that God often made a holy connection for us that was a real blessing. God is a connection expert. The other day I was given a magazine at a physiotherapist's office by the receptionist. It was a special collector's edition of the 2014 Sochi Olympics. I was surprised to read an article in it about a third cousin whom I knew but hadn't heard about for a number of years. He had won Canada's first Olympic Medal at the Sochi Winter Games."

"O God – How Great Thou Art"

CHAPTER 10

—

How To Be Happy In The 90s And 100s

How can you and I face the changes that come in old age and be happy and content? Are you prepared? Have you had to give up driving yet? Do you know the bus route to take you now? Or will your daughter or son be living with you and drive you places you need to go? Who knows what the future holds? Whatever the future holds, it may well limit you in ways you never experienced before. Are you adaptable or are you stuck in your ways and find it difficult to even think about change? We tend to think of the elderly person as frail and infirm, but do we see ourselves like that – yet? Can that be what's coming? It does not have to be like that you know.

You can start preparing for the inevitable so it does not hurt and confuse you as much. What are your good habits now; habits that will stand you in good stead later when you are ninety-plus? Number one is to make sure you have confidence in yourself. Trust yourself and others, don't be mean and resentful, even when it looks as if someone is planning to have you moved elsewhere. Always have a smile lighting up your face and a helpful hand outstretched to help another wherever you are living.

Another thing to watch is your sleep habits. If you are tired all the time you are likely to be grumpy with others. Don't let this happen to you. We need our friends in every age. Another thing to watch as you get older is how often you move around and stay active. If you are sitting all the time, your muscles will get weak and unable to move you around. Writers have identified some common characteristics that people late in life seem to have. They have identified a strong sense of purpose. They stay active and eat healthy foods (even when gluten-free like me). They go to church regularly or practice meditation privately. They also keep their friends as long as possible and relate to others in a friendly way.

Another interesting point is how real oldies don't like taking medicine. They put off taking a pill as the last thing to do. They are interested in living a healthy life and are keen on taking care of themselves. They stay independent as long as possible and enjoy a walk on the beach with their dogs. Psalm 92:14 is encouraging: "They shall still bear fruit in old age; they shall be fresh and flourishing."

See, it is the real you at work when you are trying to do something fresh and new.

Yet, there are things that are bound to happen to us and we fear them as we age. I have mentioned the fear of losing my independence already. There is also the weakening of declining health, which is bound to catch up with us sooner or later. The sad death of a loved one comes all too often in this age period and grief is exhausting. Have you had to give up your driver's licence? That really hurts. Not being able to drive your car badly affects one's sense of independence.

Finally, let me mention the one thing that affects us oldies the most – loneliness! Yes, it hurts and shows up how modern society does not have time for us any longer. When we're living alone it also affects our fears for no one is there to help us if we fall. It is very important to keep a positive attitude towards our abilities even though we are weaker and not able to do what we easily did before. I always thought my memory function was sound, until just the other week I forgot the right time for a dental appointment. My mind just had it all wrong. That was a shock to me as I always thought my thinking ability was still right on. Oh dear. What is coming next? No, don't say it. Only God really knows. The closer I get to really seeing Him affects how I read Scripture. For instance, have you ever noticed what Isaiah says about aging?

"Listen to Me, O house of Jacob, and all the remnant of the house of Israel, who have been upheld by Me from birth, who have been carried from the womb; even to old age, I am He, and even to gray hairs I will carry you! I have made, and I will bear; even I will carry, and will deliver you." (Isaiah 46: 3-4)

All of us oldies wonder if we have our feet securely in a place of rest and hope. As we journey through the eighties and nineties, to a hundred and wonder if we will really get there to a hundred, we are thankful for those who show us the way ahead and encourage us to follow in faith and trust in a higher power.

Your attitude towards yourself at every age influences your sense of well-being. When did you last have a positive thought towards something that you have done, now or in your memory? When your self-attitude is not favourable nothing looks good any more and your future is not favourable.

Take a moment now to reach way down deep and look with favour on your life. It is good now and will continue so in the future, even if death is included. Sadly, aging though, has lots of negative downsides. There is arthritis and that aching all over feeling first thing when you get up in the morning. How do you cope? It's your attitude that will get you through or hadn't you counted on that? A positive attitude is what will get you through what faces you. Well, what is your basic attitude towards aging? Do you have a positive attitude towards yourself? A friend of mine who is in her nineties wrote me some of her self-perceptions. Her attitude shows through clearly. Here is her story.

LIFE STORY OF BETTY AT AGE 92

"What do I contribute to my good health, my well-being and my general attitude to living? Many, many things: being a Christian and being supported by the Christian community are the most important. However, I have always recognized that we are responsible for how we live out our days. We can waste it away complaining, living a lifestyle that is detrimental to our body and mind or we can eat healthy and look after our body and well-being. Hence, I walk each day and enjoy God's creation since walking is part of my quiet time. I have regular healthy meals with lots of salads, fresh vegetables, fruit and protein, and mostly chicken and fish. I make all kinds of homemade soups and enjoy multigrain bread. This is important to me and it is done with thought and preparation. I enjoy shopping, planning meals, and looking for healthy foods.

"I enjoy cooking so I entertain often. At least once a week I have friends over for lunch or dinner. Not driving, they come to visit with me. I had a very serious accident five years ago and no longer drive. A gravel truck with a pup trailer blew me off the freeway. He was passing me as I was in the inside lane and his pup trailer jackknifed and hit me. I rolled over three times off the highway. I am fortunate to be alive as it gave me vertigo and it is no longer safe for me to drive. When I was able to walk alone, I learned the bus routes and now use the bus and SkyTrain to get around. I truly am very thankful that I can travel by public transportation.

"The bus also enables me to visit friends in assisted living complexes. I try to visit once a month, as I travel quite a bit, but I do make a point of visiting when I am at home. I also visit anyone from the church in the Langley Hospital and those in the palliative care unit. It is just a twenty-minute walk over to the hospital. I carry my Psalm book with me and church members find the Psalms comforting and appreciate a quiet prayer together. Taking time to visit at the hospital and visiting shut-ins keeps me busy and is very much appreciated.

"I also do what I can to be useful at Langley Church. I bake a lot for Sunday morning coffee, attend the new women's group, and I do the Internet for this group. I occasionally teach Sunday school and of course have newcomers over for lunch or dinner. I am president of British Columbia Synodical and continue to work with The Women's Missionary Society as I have been a member for over fifty years and it remains an important part of my life.

"I continue to be active, and my memory is still very good. I keep a day-timer close by and my cognitive skills get challenged by being this active. My attitude is, when problems arise, find some answers and I use my life-learned skills to cope. I pray and ask for help, but rejoice and give thanks for the many blessings I receive daily by being aware of the needs of those who do not enjoy good health and need a comforting presence."

Thanks Betty, you have given hope and encouragement to a lot of people.

CHAPTER 11

—

Ways To Reach 100

Do you really want to reach a hundred or are you just putting it on to impress someone? If you really are pushing the ultimate age and hoping to reach it, then here are some helpful ideas. I have been looking for the spark that I can see in those who reach late nineties and into their one hundreds.

First of all, are you looking after yourself? Do you come from a family with older sisters and brothers still alive or are you beating your own drum, feeling lonely and sad? Genetic history does play a part, so let us not wish for something that may not be within your grasp. Take a look at some of these suggestions and count them as your goals. One never knows what the future may bring you.

1. Do you take a good vacation? Or does your work take all your energy and leave you no time for a trip to a wonderful location where you can swim every day?

How I long for those days now, wonderful days at the beach swimming.

2. What kind of a worker are you? Are you conscientious or just want to get it done and out of there? If you are careful about what you do and fully complete it, then you are more likely to look on your life the same way. Be careful what you do and be careful to complete it, even when you are age ninety!

3. Do you smile at your neighbour and help your competent staff every day? Or are you a loner, aware only of what you must do. That attitude will hurt in the nineties when other people may well treat you the same way, ignoring you while doing what they must do.

4. Are you a friendly person, making several attempts to meet the other person's needs? This attitude will help you later when you are in the nineties. Others will notice your needs and reach out to help you help another.

5. Do you laugh a lot or frown all the time? You may need to look further than you are used to. Look deep and laugh, laugh, laugh. There is always a good reason to laugh unless you worry about hurting someone's feelings. Do you laugh with them or at them?

6. Are you happy? No? Maybe you are not the happy kind of person or did something happen years ago that wiped out your happy thoughts? One tends to remember hurtful occasions long into the nineties. Learn how to be happy. Start with not dwelling on hurtful memories. They can pull you down in the nineties.

7. Walk a lot if you can. Sure it is hard when you need a walker but try little by little to make it down the hall first, and then out the door to the street, and a little more each day.

8. What have you been doing that makes you feel your life has been worth it now that you are ninety? Do you have a life purpose that encourages you to wake up each morning in pursuit of it? If not, then think up one now. You need a reason for living.

9. Check your diet. Are you eating enough meat? How about fruits? What did you have this morning? Check that your diet is helping you live into the nineties.

10. Go to church and enjoy the togetherness with other people who feel the same way as you...loved. You need to be in a community. Don't stay by yourself in a

little room somewhere feeling sorry for yourself. That will just hasten your failure to live through the nineties.

11. Be optimistic always, even when it does not look like it will work out for the good. The way you relate to something has a lot to do with your ability to carry it through. Being optimistic means you are really trying and believe that it will work out OK.

12. Get enough sleep. Yes! Take a pill if you have to but your body needs rest to rejuvenate. You will never make it through the nineties tired all the time. It is a fact that old age cuts down your energy, weakens your muscles, and gives you a headache. But by the time you make it into the nineties your thoughts keep you awake so think more about the needs of others than on your own needs. If you must stay awake at night, spend time praying for those in need around you.

GILBERT'S LIFE STORY AT AGE 85
"What's for you won't go by you"

"I was born in Falkirk, Scotland on July 30th, 1929. I only have one sister. My mother worked in a shop but was originally a cook. My dad drove a bus or limousine for private hire. The family moved around a lot, depending what family hired Dad as their chauffeur.

"My family life was normal but at age twenty I left school for the army, round 1948-50. After my discharge, I started working in the Scottish coal survey lab. That job included surveying pits. It was hard work as I had to sometimes remove six-foot samples, but I was not too tired to go to night school where I took chemistry. This was while I was still in Scotland. At age twenty-two I took a job in Bahrain, in the Persian Gulf, refining and loading oil tankers. After staying there for seven years, I returned to Scotland where I settled from 1959 to 1961 so I could go to college to take Applied Chemistry.

"Remembering back to how my dad would not approve of the baptism of any of us children at birth, yet when I married Alma Kimm, I was finally baptised. This was years later in a Dutch Reform Church. I think I was twenty-five years of age by then. This was in the Middle East where I had taken a job just before being married.

"Alma Kimm and I were happily married in Scotland. We had two children but we had to wait sixteen years before the first child arrived. In 1961 we left for England where I took a job working shifts, analysing nylon inter-mediates. I worked in that plant until 1971. While there, I also took Chemical Engineering. Leaving ICI (Imperial

Chemical Industries) in 1971, we went to Dundee in Scotland, where I worked as refinery foreman. I stayed for three years but in 1974 I went to Saudi Arabia as a commissioning engineer for a year.

"Through all this coming and going, Alma worked as a nurse/midwife, and I as an engineer. I was busy starting new plants. Then the oil crisis in 1974 led to many contractors being laid off so I went home, and then on to London where I was offered a job in the Bahamas. Alma and I were in the Bahamas from 1975 to 1979. Finally, I came to Canada in 1979 where I was offered a job working for Ontario Hydro in heavy water plants, and then in a nuclear power plant.

"You ask why I moved around like I did. Where did I get the itch to keep moving? After thinking it over, I realised that it was obviously the example I had of my dad who also moved around a lot. My mother moved with him and today my sister also moves around a lot.

"In Ontario I worked as a nuclear operator until I finally retired. I was alone as Alma had died in 1985, so now I just kept on moving and moving, first to South Hampton, and then Owen Sound, then Elliot Lake in Northern Ontario, and finally to Kingston where my son was married and had a daughter. Finally I moved to Vancouver Island in

2004 or 2005 because my daughter in Duncan wanted me nearby.

"It sure looks like I was a drifter but I never had a day's unemployment. I was always going to a job or to family. 'Do you get restless now?' Iris asked me. I've driven across Canada four or five times, I told her. I have even gone down to the States. I have always had a position of authority and good pay. I met my current wife, Cathy, on the Internet through a dating program in 2008. She was living in Washington. We were married in 2009 and are happily settled here in Parksville on Vancouver Island.

"A year or so ago I broke my hip and cannot get around like I used to. Yes. I fell off a wee stand in the back room and get cheesed off sometimes but nothing bothers me too much. I can blow my top and it's finished. All my life I have been that way.

"My genes are involved here in my long, happy life. I never had an illness that was a problem. I only remember having blood poisoning when I was four years old. There was no penicillin then and they didn't know how to help me. Finally it gushed out my ankle. I have never sat still in my life until now. I beat poisoning in my blood system so I can beat anything now. My maternal grandfather was ninety-five when he died and my mother was age ninety-one.

"I remember getting a two-wheeled bicycle at age four and a half and had the good balance back then to ride it. My dad, driving a bus saw me half a mile from home and he sent me home.

"I went to church as a child, and then took a break as I moved around until I was married. We are settled in a local church now. When I moved to Parksville, I volunteered as a driver for SOS (Society of Organized Services). I had driven for various groups in Ontario after retiring. Back then, I was driving up to forty hours a week and one year I drove one hundred thousand kilometres. I did that for ten years or there about. Yes, I cared for others and even delivered Meals on Wheels.

"I have had a pretty good life and until I broke my hip I was helping to pay it back. After all – "What's for you won't go by you." It's all meant to be. That saying was one of my mother's quotes she used whenever something went wrong and it has stayed with me all my life."

CHAPTER 12

—

Aging And Memory Loss

There is nothing sadder than watching a loved one sink into dementia or Alzheimer's. How can one avoid this source that is debilitating the western world? What can we do to avoid it as we grow older?

A friend of mine is writing down her experiences as chaplain in a senior care facility. I am sure she will deal with this sad problem. Meanwhile, what can we do as we age to escape such a debilitating end?

Here are some suggestions:

Stay involved and as active as possible. Many people today are a new breed of seniors, living on their own, staying busy, and having a positive outlook on life.

Family is very important but don't let them do everything for you. You need to keep active and experience life's challenges during your whatever. Your arthritis may be getting worse but don't let it put you to bed. There are interesting things to do each day including taking a shower. I put my body through many exercises every day while showering. The hot water does miracles to my sore muscles.

What keeps you busy now? Keep at it and don't give up. You need to keep as active as possible.

Is your personal attitude one that others can emulate? Do other people admire you and appreciate what you can do? I can still play the organ in church when our regular organist is away and people appreciate that. You have many skills others can enjoy too. Age may slow your step but your optimism and positive attitude lengthens your days on earth.

If you are a smoker there is trouble ahead. If you get a cold and it affects your lungs, what will you do? The first step is to cut out as many smokes as you can until you are free of that burden.

Are you depressed now? Put that aside and look for something you can enjoy. Watch your favourite sports on TV or better still, attend a game or two and cheer up.

It is amazing what a happy disposition can do to your immune system. It can be strengthened when you become more positive and happier each day.

Take your troubles and worries to God. Whether you see yourself as spiritual or as Christian, there is a power that can help you. Talk to God every day and share your concerns with the Lord who understands, for He also suffered pain and discomfort.

Is your family close by? Talk with them on the phone or Skype every day and keep that connection alive. We need people close by, either physically or through the Internet, letting us know they care.

Whatever you do tomorrow just don't sit home and do nothing. If you are feeling sorry for yourself and don't care about anything anymore, then you won't make a hundred. Do all you can to be your best in every age – even into the nineties.

LIFE STORY OF RUTH AT AGE 56

"My story began on the east coast of Canada. I was born in Halifax, Nova Scotia and moved to Riverview, New Brunswick as a young child with my parents. As an only child I valued the community in the church. One of my earliest memories is walking with my mother each Sunday morning to our local church. During those early years our church was a little schoolhouse. We were part of a church plant. As I grew, so did the church and a new church building was constructed. I have many fond memories of growing up within that church community, in the Sunday school, the youth group, and then making my profession of faith and becoming a member of the church. I also remember my mother challenging me by making a distinction of faith being heart knowledge and not just head knowledge.

"Later on as a teenager, I remember going to the Synod camp, which was in Merigomish, Nova Scotia. There was a missionary there that summer who was instrumental in working out my call to church work. Since I didn't know any women ministers, I began to bargain with God by saying, "OK God, I will work in the church as anything but not as a minister." The only thing I could think of in the church that was not a minister was a secretary. My missionary friend from camp introduced me to Ewart College and at that time, the role of the deaconess. I still didn't have a clear picture of what a deaconess did but I knew it was different than that of a minister or a secretary.

"Following my studies at Ewart College and graduating with my diploma in Christian Education, my first ministry took me to St. Andrew's Presbyterian Church in Victoria, B.C. as the Director of Christian Education and Youth Worker. It was there that I met my husband and we started our family. We now have three grown children, Christa (and Yannick), Jesse, and Andrew, and one grandson, Armand.

"When the children were all in school, I started to do some freelance Christian education work which led into a shared ministry starting a new Presbyterian congregation in the Western Communities (on the outskirts of Victoria). In many ways, it reminded me a lot of my growing up years in the church plant in Riverview.

"Towards the end of that ministry I went to Vancouver School of Theology to complete my theological studies and graduated in 2006.

"My journey with memory loss though began in 2001 when the shared ministry in the Western Communities came to an end. Any period of transition like job loss brings about its own stress, but also opens the door to possibilities. When my position ended, a friend suggested that I take over the role of the chaplain in a seniors' care facility. I had zero experience or knowledge of dementia and a big part of this position was to do group spiritual therapy with residents of advanced dementia. I felt totally unprepared for this and I struggled with my purpose and the value of ministering with people who would not remember that I had even been there shortly after I left them. I quickly learned the gift of living in the present moment. I realized that the reason for being there and ministering with these individuals was to bring God's light to them, even if it was just for that moment. The reward for me in being in that moment was to see their genuine smiles every time I was on the unit and to feel their acceptance and welcome.

"One of the days that I remember most clearly is when I was doing spiritual therapy with a group of our most advanced dementia residents. I was doing a session on hearing and I was sharing with them the importance of getting eye contact with people when speaking with people who don't hear well. I had a group of residents who were slumped in their wheelchairs with their eyes shut and I had no indication that any of them were even understanding or listening to what I was saying. Then, almost as if on cue, they lifted their heads and looked directly at me. It was amazing. I called each of them by their names and they gave me the most wonderful smiles I have ever seen. I tell you this because so often I hear, 'Well, I don't go to see so and so any more. They don't remember me. It's no use.' It makes me question the purpose of why we visit. Are we visiting out of a sense of the past, our connectedness with the person, or can we somehow enter into the now of their existence? My suggestion for those of you who are struggling with your visits with a friend or a family member who has dementia is to be aware in the moment. Often you might notice a foot tapping if there is music playing, or if you dare to sing with them, they may surprise you when they sing along with every word or as they hum the tune. Music is such a great gift and it is a vehicle that I believe reaches the soul. I have been amazed how some residents who cannot tell me their name or where they have lived can sing every word of a song or join in with me in a scripture verse.

"The gift of dementia, and yes, I believe it is a gift if we take the time to look at it, is the present moment. The problem is that we live in a very fast-paced world most of the time. We are either living in our past remembering what it used to be like or striving hard to do things for a future, in the hope of what things might be. But we rarely take the time to enjoy the present moment. In my experience, there are two groups of people who have grasped the gift of the present moment – the very young children and seniors. We have a program at my work where we bring very young children in to interact with the elderly and it is a special moment indeed. There is something very special when these two age groups have the opportunity to interact.

"In my work as a chaplain I have been amazed and blessed by the care of family members. I have seen family members who come every day or every second day, and have created wonderful memories with their loved ones. Their enduring love 'for better or for worse, in sickness and in health,' continues to amaze me. One particular husband arrives every day and when I ask him how he is, he always looks up at me with a smile and says, 'I'm with my girl.' Enough said. Another family member has said, 'It takes a village. This is my village.'

"Facing a health challenge as we age is never easy. For some, they are caring for their loved ones while facing their own health challenges. One family member says, 'Sometimes it was hard coming to visit when I was feeling poorly, but I knew she needed me more than I needed my bed. In other words, Mom kept me going and now my new friends are doing the same.' Now that her mother is no longer here, she continues to come while her health allows it, to volunteer.

"In a recent study, the Alzheimer Society has stated that physical activity may be a significant factor in reducing the risk of developing dementia. Going out for a walk once a day and then increasing the distance a bit at a time can have a major effect for us as we age. I spoke with a lady a while ago who was having some physical problems, so much actually that she was being told she would have to be in a wheelchair soon. She read in a magazine that walking was good for her health so she decided to give it a try. At first, she only made it past a couple of houses and back, then she made it further until she could make it around the block and then further. She went on to walking ten-kilometer race events, and then half marathon events. Now that she is in her eighties she is still walking and doing ten kilometer race events and is a great spokesperson for health and well-being.

"Other aspects that may help in reducing the risk of developing dementia are eating healthy foods and keeping our minds active. There is a wealth of information these days about the types of food we should be eating and ones that we should stay away from so I am not going to dwell on diet in this short chapter. As far as keeping our minds active, there are all sorts of different puzzles like cross-words, word search, and Sudoku that help us to think and keep mentally active. We can also do things like memorizing phone numbers or Bible verses or doing mental math instead of relying on things like calculators. Besides physical activity and keeping our minds active we also need to feed our spirit. I always begin our spiritual therapy sessions with our residents by asking them how their spirit is. It would be a good practice for all of us to come in touch with how our spirit is each day. What nurtures your spirit? Perhaps it's a walk by the ocean or near the mountains or a meadow. Perhaps it is a walk with a special friend or time alone to meditate. Perhaps it is doing something for someone else. It is a proven fact that volunteering your time to help someone else can lift your spirit.

"Besides being a chaplain I am also the coordinator of Volunteer Services. I often hear from the volunteers that they get more out of their work than what they think they give to others. If you're not feeling good about yourself or what's going on, one of the best things you can do is just get up and go out and do something with or for someone else. It will give you a different perspective on life and a spiritual facelift. So as a preventative measure for reducing the risk of developing dementia, make sure you are nurturing your body, mind, and spirit. It all works together. This goes for all of us in every stage of life but especially as we age and enter the autumn years of life. What are the things you are doing to nurture your physical body, your mind, and your spirit?

"My personal involvement with dementia began when my mother was diagnosed with vascular dementia. Working in the field of health care in a senior's care facility prepared me to some degree, but the reality of having a loved one needing care was completely different. I had to shift gears from being the professional to the family member. I became instantly immersed in all the emotions that every family member experiences. I believe it has given me new insight in my work as a professional. I still say today that the hardest thing I have ever had to do is place my mother in a care facility. As a family member, you always want to do the best thing for your loved one and be the one to care for them. It took me a while to understand that the best I could do for my mother and for myself was to place her in the care of others who could look after her needs 24 hours a day around the clock. While in care, I watched my mother sink deeper into the dementia and then lose her mobility, which was a double blow.

"I remember speaking to one of the men at our church who had just lost his wife to Alzheimer's. When I told him about my mother, I remember the way he looked at me and he just said two words, 'Visit lots.' He understood what it meant to love someone with dementia and he had walked down the path I was just beginning. He knew how I would feel when it was over.

"The most telling mark for me with my mother's dementia was the day that she called me to her side in the care home and she told me that she 'thought' she loved me. My heart broke. At what stage does a person not remember that they love someone, but something deep down in their soul tells them that this is a person who they love? I wanted to cry out but instead I held my mother's hand and told her that I 'knew' she loved me and assured her that I loved her.

"The verse that came to my mind was Isaiah 49:15, 'Can a woman forget her nursing child, or show no compassion for the child of her womb? Even these may forget, yet I will not forget you.'

"Another instance with my mother in the care facility was when her care worker said to her as he pointed to me, 'Do you know who this is?'

"She looked at me and back at him and said, 'Of course silly, that's my daughter … and you are my son.'

"Living with someone with dementia is living in the moment. We value every moment we have with our loved one and make memories together any way we can.

"There will be many moments where patience will be needed. Sometimes we will want to reach out and help our loved one, but sometimes it is more important for our loved one to do for themselves. I remember a time in the care facility when we were going to go in the elevator. In this particular care facility they had designed a security measure that to use the elevator you needed to put in a stick in a hole to push the button. My mother figured she could use her pinky finger to do this. Well, on this particular day I quickly grabbed the stick to push the button. This was the first time that my mother ever swore at me. This was one of the last things that she felt she still had control over and she could do herself and I took it away from her. I never did that again. It may take them longer to do something but it is very important that we have patience with them and let them do things as long as they can.

"I'm not sure when the reversal of roles happened but it does happen and it is bound to happen. They are our parent but at some point as the caregiver you become the parent of the parent but the parent is always your parent. We need to treat them with the same patience and love that they have given to us throughout our lives. We can't argue with them or tell them what they are doing is wrong because in their mind it is right. We can't treat them like a child even if they are acting like a child. We just need to continue to love them, support them, and accept them for who they are. And as each day brings a new challenge you will learn to walk together.

"I remember one son who used to come and visit his mother. He was what some of us would refer to as 'the black sheep in the family.' When he returned home after being away from his family for many years, he was told that his mother had died. Perhaps in some people's minds, that is what happens when someone travels down the road to dementia. Anyway, many years later this son discovered that his mother had not died but was in a care facility. He was a very faithful son. He came every week to visit his mother even though she did not recognize him as her son.

She thought he was her boyfriend and they would hold hands together during each visit. He would come on the day that he knew I was doing a spiritual therapy group on her floor. He was not a church-going person but our spiritual therapy group became his 'church' as long as his mother was with us. He learned the value of living in the moment.

"I remember as a student doing a research paper on the topic of spiritual care for someone with dementia. Of course, this was way before my journey had started with my mother, but even back then I was struck by the title of an article I found in the library. It was entitled "The Never-ending Funeral." I thought that described dementia so well because with the loss of memories the family loses that person bit by bit. So with all the losses I felt as a daughter of someone with dementia, I thought that when the time came for my mother's death I would not feel grief but relief. I was wrong. My grief was intense. Yes, there was relief because the journey of the road called dementia was finally over for my mother but intense grief because she was gone. What gave me hope and healing was our common faith that she was in the arms of her Saviour and one day we would meet again and enjoy an eternity together.

"If you are reading this chapter as a person who is caring for someone with dementia, or if you have some of the signs yourself of dementia, I hope that my experience has helped you a bit. I encourage you to reach out to people who can give you support and walk with you. There are agencies that can help you to navigate through this difficult road. The first step will be to see your doctor and be assessed for services. There is a wide range of services available. Your doctor will be able to help you find other resources as well. The Alzheimer's Society has many excellent resources and support groups in most areas. Don't be afraid to ask questions. There are people around who can help you through this.

"My final word of wisdom is to remember the love you shared and hold on to that love. If there is one thing that will break through the haze of the dementia, it is love. My mother recognized it in me when she did not know me. 'These three remain: faith, hope and love. But the greatest of these is love.' 1 Corinthians 13:13."

CHAPTER 13

—

Afraid Of Aging

If we are really honest with each other, what would we say? Try this answer for size. No, I am not afraid of aging; I am looking forward to the thrill of telling everyone I have reached a hundred! Does that fit you? Most will say, "NO." They are really afraid of aging.

However, if we are just in our eighties and nineties what then would we say to this question? Would we still give a negative answer? "I am not afraid." Or would we have to admit, "Yes, I am afraid of aging. I am not looking forward to getting weaker. I won't be able to drive the car. Now I am already having eye trouble, and I am not able to stand up on my own without help. I am not able to live alone any more either. Gosh, I can't even cook my meals now." Shucks!

There is another negative thought, a painful one at that – having all one's teeth out! See what's ahead of you.

There are a lot of disadvantages in living beyond seventy-five. Would we really choose to live so long?

There are also several other faculties that start to deteriorate. One of the saddest is the lack of feeling our emotions really moving us. When we were younger our emotions got triggered. We really felt joy and sadly, we really felt grief. Now as we age, these emotions slacken and we don't even remember how we felt years ago when we were feeling the joy of discovering something beautiful. Now when I listen to beautiful music it tends to move me to tears instead of joy. Our feelings are not top notch any more. It is really very sad not to feel something at its best any more. I really sense this loss when listening to music.

One big need is the support of family members as one grows older. If family is far away one has to at least talk with them on a regular basis. The younger generation is so busy these days. The cultural demands that keep things rolling along must be met. There are business and other demands, and family is never just sitting back and enjoying life these days. Face it! They don't have time for you and if they did the need to look after you makes their demands sound bossy because they are in a hurry. Forgive and forget and keep growing.

What about loss of independence? Can you still take care of yourself? The thought of having strangers in to look after you can be frightening. Is your health stable or do you get weaker each day as you look out at another gloomy morning? At least, if you can still get out of bed you can still rise up with a smile, can't you? Even getting dressed sometimes becomes hard when you can't bend down. Taking a shower or getting into the tub is no longer a thrill but is a possible distraction as you could fall and break a leg or break something else.

One really big worry these days is running out of money. You have always tried to be prudent and not waste your money, but who has your funds now? This could put a real worry on your loved ones. Also one of the hardest things to bear as you age is the death of a loved one. More of one's friends and relatives are passing away and you are still left. It is truly sad. One has a real sense of loss. Who can take your loved ones place? Can anyone?

I think we would agree that the main reason for fearing aging is the possible loss of mental faculties and loss of the ability to perform the usual daily tasks because you cannot remember what they are!

Every day is dicey, for it could trap you into doing something stupid and your life would never be the same. May I suggest that you pray each day, asking God to guide you in all you do so that you can feel safe and enjoy each day through the eighties, nineties, and a hundreds? It is true that God will see you through each day if you ask Him. He will bring things together in surprisingly helpful ways. This is the work of the Holy Spirit and He is really good at it. I speak from experience.

LIFE STORY OF DOROTHY AT AGE 91

"I was born in Halifax, Nova Scotia on November 14th 1923. My mother was fifth generation Nova Scotian and her forbearers came from the Boston area. My father was originally from England. I spent my first three years in Nova Scotia and then moved to Britain. I grew up there until the war broke out while we were visiting my mother's family and we were forced to stay in Canada. Later we moved to Ottawa, where my father joined the war effort by forming the Department of Goods and Services. I was an only child and therefore the focus of attention by my fabulous parents. I was sick a lot, first with tuberculosis, and later faced death from pneumonia as well as pleurisy. I was never scared for I was led to believe by my mother that I had an angel always with me. I was fortunate to have a doctor who believed in natural remedies and I was cured. The doctor's name was Dr. Grantly Dick-Read, who became very famous as the first to write a book on Natural Childbirth.

"While in Ottawa, I attended Ottawa Ladies College. Among the students were a number of relatives of the queen, who had been forced to stay in Canada because of the war. After graduation I went to work at the main branch of the Bank of Montreal. Among the many interesting customers was Princess Juliana of the Netherlands. My biggest challenge came when I was asked to become a teller and was presented with my cash box, on top of which was a large gun. I stated that if this was necessary to the position I would have to turn it down. After a lengthy discussion by management it was decided that the gun could be dispensed with. I always spoke up for myself as my father had taught me. In a very short space of time all tellers' guns were gone!

"I was approached to enlist in the British Army, but Mother was very unwell and I was concerned that if I joined I might be posted elsewhere. I did not wish to leave my mother. Instead I went to work as a civilian with the British Army. I had many wonderful experiences and met interesting people from many countries. I was asked to open an office for the army in Montreal with staff. My assistant Violet and I went together and opened that office. One night there was a big bang on our bedroom door at the hotel. It was our captain, who ordered us to be up, dressed, and in the lobby in ten minutes. We got dressed and went with the captain to the docks where goods were being unloaded from trains from the United States, onto Russian freighters, which were bound for Britain. These were military supplies, which Roosevelt had agreed to send to Britain under the lend lease program that he had arranged with Churchill. Without this arrangement England would undoubtedly have fallen.

"The weather was freezing cold and wet, but men on the Russian ship gave us trousers to protect us from the cold. Once again back in Ottawa, I was asked to open another office for the British Army, this time in Washington DC. My memory of Washington was of heat and humidity.

"By this time, I had become engaged to my husband-to-be. Leslie was a naval officer and he had been at sea for some time. He was aboard a navy vessel whose function was to launch depth charges with the hope of destroying German submarines. My parents, especially my father, were not happy with my choice. I had made my commitment to this handsome naval officer and went through with the marriage. When we were driving away on our honeymoon, I looked back to see my father crying.

"I was blessed by the birth of my son Alan, but there were problems with the marriage. One of the many problems was how Leslie handled money. He hid the fact that he had money from me, and his discharge from the navy. Then he had me pay for clothing suitable to find employment.

"After we moved to Montreal, where we bought a house using my money as a down payment, the marriage continued to deteriorate. I stayed with Leslie until after his mother Helen passed away. I was very fond of Helen and did not wish to hurt her by leaving her son. After she passed away I moved to a small apartment over a nearby pharmacy so I could be close to Alan. With the help of a detective I found out that Leslie was having an affair with his secretary.

"By that time I had met and fallen in love with Ossie (Osbourne), and after our divorces became final we decided to marry. We had difficulty finding a United Church minister who was willing to marry divorcees, but we finally did and were off to Bermuda for our honeymoon, with I would add, my parent's full blessing! Sadly, two years after our marriage, I had to have surgery for cancer. As a result we were unable to have children. Fortunately our love for one another got us past this sadness.

"After travelling to the west, Ossie and I fell in love with the coast. We decided to move there but business opportunities were limited. The government had a business development branch and with their backing we decided to open a carpet mill in Kelowna. We had to supply investment dollars as well and it was a huge challenge for Ossie to find these funds. Though smart, he was a very shy man and he had to accomplish this task on his own as no one in those days would listen to a woman. He managed to raise a million dollars, which was an incredible amount of money at that time and the mill was built.

"As the years went by, the business grew to a point where we needed more capitol to expand. Unfortunately the government, through the same development department, partnered us with investors who proved to be dishonest and as a result the business failed and we lost it all. We then moved to Vancouver with my father who had stayed with us through everything. With his help, we obtained a loan, which allowed us to start another business whole-saling very high quality fabrics and carpets. Initially we opened a small showroom but as the business grew we moved to a large, six-thousand square-foot showroom on Beatty Street. Finally we had a thriving business until the 1980s when there was a huge economic downturn. As a result of both suppliers and customers going bankrupt all around us, our business also failed. However I take great pride in saying that we did not declare bankruptcy.

"I managed to pay off all our debts, a task I had to accomplish on my own, because the situation had caused Ossie's health to collapse and he had taken two strokes and was in hospital. He finally had nine strokes before he passed away. Before Ossie's health completely deteriorated, we had several good years of travelling across North America, pulling our small travel trailer. Many people thought me mad travelling with a man who had been so ill, but I decided we were not going to sit around waiting for my love to die but enjoy what time we had left together. I have never regretted that decision.

"During this difficult time I met and was mentored by a brilliant man, Dr. Bob Owen, who introduced me to health promoting products. Now in my sixties and in poor health myself, introduction to this new world not only caused our health (Ossie's and mine) to improve, but it allowed me to reach out and help literally thousands of others. I went on to build a very large network business when in my mid-seventies. This provided the much-needed funds to give my love the best possible care in his final days.

"Yes, God's angel has been with me, even when things were really bad. I am not afraid of death myself, but I was heartbroken to lose Ossie. I wanted to hold on to him as we had such a wonderful life together and a marriage that other people dream about. I finally had to give him permission to go and his passing was peaceful. He went to be with his brothers at the nineteenth hole of God's golf course.

"At that time, my adopted son Blake and I were living in a townhouse in Surrey. Blake had come into our lives when he came to our showroom looking for fabrics for his design jobs. Ossie always said that boy is coming in to visit his mother. We had moved into the townhouse in hopes of bringing Ossie home from long-term care but it was not meant to be. After Ossie passed we decided we did not want to stay in the house. I moved back to my lovely mobile home and Blake headed to Qualicum Beach. After I was told my eyesight would fail, Blake asked if the cat (Toto) and I would move to Qualicum Beach and live with him.

"These days I am limited to the things I can do physically, but fortunately am still mentally fit, enabling me to share my knowledge and help others to restore their health. I am aware that approaching age ninety-one, the Creator still has work for me to do and I will continue until He calls me home to be with my angels."

CHAPTER 14

—

What The Bible Says About Aging

Where does one start? If we look in Genesis or the New Testament verses, there are so many that speak of aging. I will begin with some verses that speak to me personally. After all, that is how the Bible speaks to us – it gets personal! Psalm 91:16 says, "With long life I will satisfy them and show them my salvation." What is the long life meant here? How many years make a long life? When you look at the passing years from earth's stance a few years ago it could mean forty to eighty years. But now look at human life from God's stance. As Peter said in 2 Peter 3: 8, "A thousand years is like a day."

The Bible presents growing old as normal. It is a natural part of life and involves increased wisdom and experience. "Grey hair is a crown of splendour, it is attained by a righteous life." That is what Proverbs 16:31 says. But as we grow older, things start to wane: less energy, muddled thinking, hesitant walking etc. The hope of making a real mark in the world grows dim. We haven't made a name for ourselves, and have no lasting legacy that will make the papers when we die. (Ecclesiastes 2)

Solomon gives us some hope that people, you and I, will grow wiser in the use of their God-given portion before they die. (Psalm 90:12) In the New Testament these concepts can be found portrayed vividly in Jesus' parables of the ten virgins, the talents (Matthew 25), the two sons (Matthew 21:28 – 32) and the unjust steward (Luke 16: 1 – 13.)

Knowing that God has given us this portion called life, we should take joyful advantage of all our gifts bestowed on us at birth by God's grace. Let us daily thank Him for the talents, wisdom, and opportunities in life we have had before all opportunity to do so ceases. Life has meaning in our God-given purpose, which is only fulfilled when we take advantage of the new life given us in Jesus Christ. Read 2 Corinthians 5:10 and be thankful as we realise that our portion was never uneven but carefully bestowed on us.

If we are looking at a long life coloured by the fear of dementia, we read of the renewing of the mind in Romans 12:2. You want to read the rest? Here it is: "Do not conform to the patterns of the world, but be transformed by the renewing of your mind." I tried that with my friend Dorothy as she sank lower and lower into the gloom of dementia. Sharing with her never conformed to the modern patterns all around her. During her life Dorothy was a firm believer in the Lord Jesus Christ. He did not desert her at the end.

What if life seems boring as days stretch on confined to a bed in a home care facility? Would Philippians 1: 6 speak to us? "Being confident of this that He who began a good work in you will carry it on to completion until the Day of Christ Jesus." Is there something you need to do yet? Would this Scripture verse bless you with a new thought? "I still have the strength to write this for God has His hand in it helping me complete it before carrying me home to Heaven."

As one gets older, especially when one is getting weaker, it is the belief that life here is a walk with Jesus that keeps us going. He holds our hands. Having Jesus beside us gives us strength, for we walk in the shade of His strength. Just look how God used a very old lady to bring about His Divine will. Yes Elizabeth, John the Baptist's mother, was a very old women way beyond bearing a child yet she did. (Luke 1:7)

Can we still remember back to the day we accepted Jesus as our Saviour? Can our memories write a history of how Jesus has carried us through to the present old age? If not, maybe you need to accept Him again. Why not do so quietly in your room so He will stay by your side as you go through these hard last years on earth. Read Colossians 3: 9,10, 11-17 and pray. He is here now with you. "Now you must rid yourself of all such things as these: anger, rage, malice, slander and filthy language from your lips and put on the new self which is being renewed in knowledge in the image of the Creator." I cannot think of a better way than this to get old, old, old.

Job 12:12 is one of my favourite verses, helping me stand up and try again. "Is not wisdom found among the aged? Does not long life bring understanding?" I have found among the aged a friendship that goes beyond what I can do for them and settles on just their love for me.

Does a person's sinful life; the constant disobedience, the lack of friendship as this fast paced culture leaves no time for family, does it mean that there is no time for Jesus too? Ephesians 6:2-3 says, "Honour your father and mother so it may go well with you." The family starts with mother and father. What happened back then may need to be taken to the Lord as it can affect your inner soul all your life into old age, causing deep sorrow. Jeremiah 29:11 reminds us, "For I know the plans I have for you, declares the Lord. Plans to prosper you not to harm you, plans to give you hope and a future." So we do not lose heart.

"Though our outer self is wasting away, our inner self is being renewed day by day." 2 Corinthians 4: 16.

Why not take a look again at a wonderful verse about aging. Isaiah 46: 4, 5 says, "Even to your old age and gray hairs I am He! I am He who will sustain you. I have made you and I will carry you; I will sustain you and I will rescue you. To whom will you compare me or count me equal?" There! Isn't that a great verse about our God? He loves you!

CHAPTER 15

—

Facing Death

If there is anything that senior oldies are really afraid of it is this – DEATH! It even looks horrible on the line above. It is the big unknown. We can deny this fear all **we** want to but eventually it will catch up with us. At this age as an oldie senior we have all experienced a loved one, a friend, a relative dying. We are not immune to the sadness and the horror of facing something we cannot help much. If God is not part of your life then who or what do you turn to now as you shiver and ache, watching someone die in front of you? Is there a good way to die? What is the worst way to die? Dementia?

For the last two years I spent many days at the side of my partner Dorothy. She had been a real friend to me for over twenty years as we retired together, bought a Recreational Vehicle and travelled everywhere. I loved the evening campfire with those sticky foods we all know so well. We loved the ocean in Mexico and I can still hear the birds singing as we swam in the local pool at the close of day. Now she lay there in bed with dementia, gone from me, her eyes open but dead. There was no spark left in her. I prayed with her often while holding her hand but the only time she woke up was when the therapy doggy jumped in her lap.

Yes, I have watched many people die of all ages but dying from dementia is hard to watch and listen to. Dorothy would scream down the hall as I left. I had never seen Dorothy so angry. So looking back now, I wonder if I looked at her with my own feelings – of shock and sadness, but also because of my own fear of death. I am aware of all our needs during these oldie senior years to prepare ourselves for death, that of a loved one, and of ourselves.

I personally would prefer to die from a stroke but I have no control over that, only God has that. To help one go through the shadow of death without fear, we need to go to the Bible. There is good reason Psalm 23 is so loved as it says, "Even though I walk through the valley of the shadow of death I will fear no evil, for you are with me." God goes through the shadow of death with us. He takes us by the hand and walks us through with love and confidence. There is nothing to really fear, all is just shadows. Yes, we do want to know what is coming next around the corner as bit by bit our bodies deteriorate, but we need not fear what is coming. All is in the shadows, that lonely place where we stand alone and are lost and fearful of what is coming next.

I can give you all kinds of Scripture verses to help you here but what you really want is to hear God speaking to you in the quiet of the lonely night. He says, "Do not be afraid for I am with you!" That inner voice can reach us with different words but His presence is what helps pick us up as He carries us through. That is exactly how it happens.

I wonder, in this secular day and age, how people face death without Jesus nearby. Do you have a spiritual bent? Do you take moments of your day and look for a spiritual truth? As more and more grandchildren and great-grandchildren leave the church their families attended, I wonder if any of you are looking for spiritual truths, looking for something that puts human life into perspective. Perhaps you believe in Heaven, or maybe you only believe in the best life can offer here and now. But what happens to you as you move beyond this earthly realm? What do you hold on to? Sure, you and your loved ones have led good lives. You have also been good parents and friends for the needy, but who is reaching out to you now as you kneel beside the bed and watch your loved one slip away?

You have reached that special time when God draws near you. Open up to Him now before it is too late. As you pray for help and comfort, the peace He offers you is amazing and flows through you from top to bottom, through your heart and mind. God does care. When His Son took human form, He died to save us all. All we need to do is accept that He is real, giving us a wonderful salvation that will take us triumphantly home to Heaven in that farewell day. Why have we been so fearful? It need not be a day of horror, but a day of great love as the Spirit of our Creator flows through us with peace. Wonderful! We are going home! I don't fear that anymore. I look forward to it. Will you come with me?

RAYMONDE'S LIFE STORY AT AGE 89

"I was born on April 25th, 1925 in the town of Lévis, Quebec. My mother already had three children from a previous marriage (sadly, she was widowed at the young age of 28) and together with my younger brother, we formed a very loving family. I had quite a happy and uneventful adolescence. As a young adult, I became involved in different youth movements. I also tried many things such as singing, piano, drawing, and painting.

My younger brother, three years younger than me, had always wanted to become a sailor just like our father. While working on a ship one day, he fell and drowned. He was only eighteen years old. I fell into a deep depression. My father, heartbroken and feeling partly responsible for his son's death, having introduced his son to a life on ships, died three years later of a heart attack. With time, healing took place and life went on.

I had many friends, boys and girls, and in particular two male friends. These friendships could potentially have led to more serious relationships. However, what I did not know at the time is that there was someone else from very far away whom God knew was destined for me. Wonderful moments lay ahead. In 1958, my older sister Gisèle had just lost her husband. She decided to rent a room to a university student to make some extra money. She received news that the only student who was still looking for a room to rent was a young man from Alberta. He was coming to Quebec City's Laval University to learn French. She agreed to accept him as a tenant as he seemed very well-mannered and pleasant. My sister asked me to come over to translate as she needed to communicate with this young man. That is how I first met Hugh Myers. As I would often visit my sister, I became more and more acquainted with Hugh. I happily served as his tour guide showing him around Quebec City. He returned home to Alberta for a while during which time we corresponded regularly.

Hugh returned to Quebec the following year for another course and that is when we started making plans for our future. We were married on December 26th, 1959. Who could ever have imagined such a thing, so far away from each other and coming together like this! I cannot help but believe that it was a part of God's plan all along. We always respected the vows we exchanged and grew old together in peace and happiness until the death of my dear Hugh in November 2012. We had been together for fifty-three years.

Our greatest accomplishments during our marriage were our three children. We experienced the loss of our first-born child, Elisabeth, when she was only six months old. This tragic event was truly a test of our faith and we each grieved in our own way. Together we somehow survived and were later blessed with the arrivals of our son Stephen and our daughter Grace.

When our children were older I became involved as a volunteer. I spent many years helping drive people to appointments, driving for Meals On Wheels, etc. I then started doing volunteer work for the Institute for the Blind. For fifteen years I spent one day a week reading for the blind employees of the Institute who would then translate the reading section into Braille. This was a wonderful experience and I looked forward to my volunteer day every week. Despite their handicap, the people I worked with had an optimism, a real joy in life that was truly inspiring. I really felt that they were giving me a gift rather than the other way around.

There were of course other sad times in my life as other close family members passed away. Our family life continued to be filled with many happy moments. Our children have always given us back the love and devotion we gave them. They continue to do so with me as I age alone and it is thanks to them, their spouses, and my two grandchildren, that I am able to go through this phase of my life feeling safe and for the most part serene.

I do experience moments of sadness when I think of my dear husband, but I know he is helping me as I feel his spirit visiting me during these difficult times. We recently lost Hugh's only sister, Dorothy, and because of risks to my health, I was not able to attend her funeral in British Columbia. I felt very alone the day of the funeral; I so wanted to be there for Dorothy and for Hugh. I decided to go for a little walk around my apartment building. Normally, I can only walk for a few feet before needing to rest. However, on that day I was able to go around the whole building without feeling fatigued. To me, this was a sure sign that the spirits of Dorothy and Hugh were with me as they had both always enjoyed their walks and they were now with me to support me. Therefore, I truly feel that our loved ones do live on within us.

That being said, I have different emotions regarding my own death. There are times when I feel quite afraid of death: how it will happen, the unknown of the afterlife, etc. At times, things can seem dark and hopeless. Despite all of this, I am able to wake up day after day with a renewed feeling of peace, hope, and acceptance. Finally, I have heard it said that aging is a privilege and I think that. At eighty-nine years of age, I am able to embrace such a saying, thanks to the love

that surrounds me and the grace of God.

CONCLUSION

Living by Faith

"For this reason we never become discouraged. Even though our physical being is gradually decaying, yet our spiritual being is renewed day after day. And this small and temporary trouble we suffer will bring us a tremendous and eternal glory, much greater than the trouble. "For we fix our attention, not on things that are seen, but on things that are unseen. What can be seen lasts only for a time, but what cannot be seen lasts forever."

2 Corinthians 4:16-18 Good News Translation (GNT)

MEMORIAL

This book is written in memory of my spiritual sister Dorothy, who died recently from dementia and its effects on her body and mind.

Dorothy is with the Lord and may be watching me and our storytellers as we share what life is all about – living to His glory.

About the Author

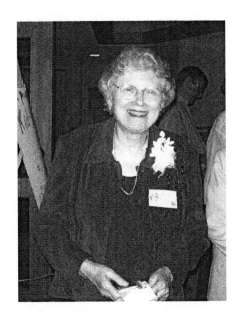

Rev. Iris M. Ford is a retired Presbyterian minister living on beautiful Vancouver Island, British Columbia. She has worked all over Canada sharing in the lives of many people from coast to coast, serving the Lord and helping people cope with life's difficulties. She has written ten books and this one has really grabbed her attention. Iris says, "This book is her last" - so she says now. But it is fascinating, drawing people of all ages into its scope. We are all aging.

CPSIA information can be obtained at www.ICGtesting.com
Printed in the USA
LVOW06*2053190215

427619LV00001B/7/P